*Interim Report:*
*Proposed Recommendations for Action*
# A National
# Public Health Initiative
# on Diabetes and Women's Health

**Acknowledgements:**
*We would like to thank Susan Baker Toal for her expert assistance in compiling and editing this document; and Odette E. Colón, Graphic Specialist in support of OD/IRM, CDC, for her creativity and graphic design skill. We would also like to thank the Association of State and Territorial Health Officials (ASTHO) for their assistance in printing this interim report.*

**Sponsored by:**

Centers for Disease Control and Prevention
American Diabetes Association
American Public Health Association
Association of State and Territorial Health Officials

# CONTENTS

# EXECUTIVE SUMMARY

Diabetes is a serious public health issue affecting more than 17 million Americans, more than half of whom are women. With the increasing life span of women and the rapid growth of minority racial and ethnic populations in the United States (who are hardest hit by the diabetes burden), the number of women at high risk for diabetes and its complications will continue to increase, placing added demands on the health care delivery system and on other sectors of society. The estimated cost of diabetes to the United States for direct health care and other indirect expenditures is about $100 billion annually.

In 2000, the Centers for Disease Control and Prevention (CDC) established the National Public Health Initiative on Diabetes and Women's Health, which has three phases. In Phase I, *Diabetes & Women's Health Across the Life Stages: A Public Health Perspective* was prepared. This report, published in 2001, examines the issues that make diabetes a serious public health problem for women; analyzes the epidemiologic, psychosocial, socioeconomic, and environmental dimensions of women and diabetes; and discusses the public health implications. In Phase II, the information contained in the Phase I report was converted into an interim report containing recommendations for needed strategies, policies, disease tracking, and research to improve the lives of women diagnosed with or at risk for diabetes. Phase III will involve preparing and implementing the National Public Health Action Plan on Diabetes and Women's Health. This final phase of the Initiative will translate the recommendations into concrete operational programs and policies for relevant agencies and organizations.

This interim report culminates Phase II and was prepared jointly by four cosponsoring organizations: CDC, the American Diabetes Association (ADA), the American Public Health Association (APHA), and the Association of State and Territorial Health Officials (ASTHO). The purpose of this report is to offer priority recommendations for responding to diabetes as a prominent public health issue for women and to garner the attention of policy makers, public health professionals, other advocates for women's issues, researchers, and the general public. In particular, this document provides recommendations for persons charged with making decisions and affecting policies related to diabetes and women's health.

This interim report outlines the vision and goals for the National Public Health Initiative on Diabetes and Women's Health, guiding principles, a public health framework, and a life stage approach for addressing diabetes and women's health. These life stages are the adolescent years (ages 10-17 years), the reproductive years (ages 18-44 years), the middle years (ages 45-64 years), and the older years (ages 65 years and above). Many of the recommendations for public health action pertain to all women, regardless of life stage; others are life stage-specific. While the emphasis is specifically on women's health, adopting and implementing many of the recommendations will improve the health and well-being of men and families as well.

1

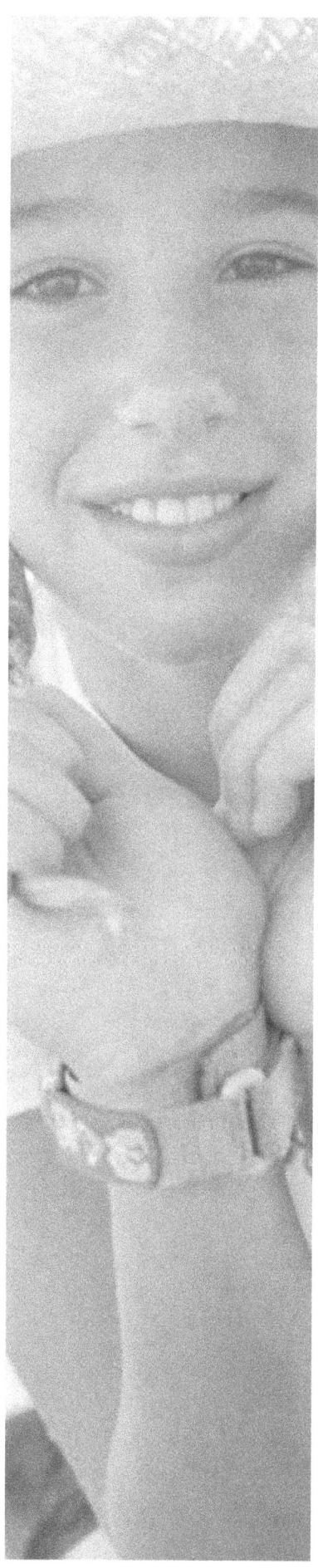

The ultimate vision is a nation in which:
- diabetes among women is prevented whenever possible,
- early diagnosis and appropriate management of diabetes among women is promoted across the life stages,
- the occurrence of complications from diabetes among women is prevented, delayed, or minimized, and
- women at risk for diabetes are provided the family and community support needed to prevent diabetes and its complications.

The underlying principles support:
- a public health approach,
- collaboration within and between multiple sectors of society,
- consideration for the unique needs of different life stages among racial, ethnic, religious, and cultural groups,
- full engagement of women and grassroots organizations,
- shared accountability by state and community leaders,
- actions based on sound research,
- measurable outcomes with which to evaluate progress, and
- sustainability of strategies and policies over time.

Several key strategy and policy recommendations pertaining to women of all ages call for:
- strengthening advocacy on behalf of women with or at risk of diabetes,
- increasing awareness among the general public about the seriousness and preventability of diabetes in women,
- expanding community-based health promotion education, activities, and incentives for women of all ages in a wide variety of settings, such as schools, workplaces, senior centers, churches, civic organizations, and others,
- integrating diabetes messages and prevention activities within the larger context of chronic disease prevention and health promotion,
- enhancing community development policies and practices (including "smart growth" initiatives and empowerment zones) that promote safe environments for physical activity,
- increasing availability and access to healthy food choices for all sectors of the population,
- supporting policies and programs in schools and workplaces that respect the health-related needs of their female students and employees, particularly women with or at risk for diabetes,
- increasing the capacity of community programs to develop and disseminate "best practices" and lessons learned,
- assuring access to trained health care providers who offer quality services to prevent and manage diabetes among women of all ages, and
- expanding public and private health insurance packages to provide adequate coverage for preventive care, including health promotion, health and nutritional education, physical activity, self-management, and screening for complications among women diagnosed with diabetes.

# BACKGROUND

## The Diabetes Burden Among Women

Diabetes mellitus is a disease caused by the body's inability to produce or properly use insulin, a hormone required to convert sugar, starches, and other food into energy. There are three main types of diabetes. Type 1 diabetes is a disease in which the body does not produce any insulin. This form occurs most often in children and young adults and accounts for 5%-10% of all cases of diabetes. Persons with type 1 diabetes must take daily insulin injections to stay alive. Type 2 diabetes is a metabolic disorder resulting from the body's inability to make enough, or properly use, insulin. Type 2 diabetes is the most common form of the disease, accounting for 90%-95% of diabetes. Primary interventions involve a healthy diet and physical activity. The third type, gestational diabetes, is a form of glucose intolerance that is diagnosed in some women during pregnancy. Treatment is required to normalize maternal blood glucose levels and avoid complications for the infant. After pregnancy, 5%-10% of women with gestational diabetes are diagnosed with type 2 diabetes, and 20%-50% develop type 2 diabetes in the next 5-10 years.

Diabetes can be associated with serious complications and even premature death. The burden of diabetes for women is unique because the disease can affect both mothers and their unborn children. With the increasing life span of women, the rapid growth of minority racial and ethnic populations in the United States (who are hardest hit by the diabetes burden), delayed initiation of childbearing, and the recent increase in new cases of diabetes among younger women in their teen years, the number of women at high risk for diabetes and its complications will continue to increase. These trends will place added demands on the health care delivery system and other sectors of society associated with determinants of health such as political, environmental, and civic entities. Although researchers have not yet identified the cause of diabetes, they have concluded that both genetic and environmental factors, such as obesity and lack of physical activity, play a major role. Lifestyle interventions designed to promote weight loss, increase physical activity, and improve diet can significantly reduce and delay the incidence of type 2 diabetes among persons at high risk for the disease.

### *Diabetes Is a Serious and Growing Public Health Problem*
- By the year 2050, the number of persons with diagnosed diabetes is projected to rise from 11 million to 29 million.
- More than 17 million Americans have diabetes.
- One million new cases of diabetes are diagnosed each year.
- Diabetes costs the United States about $100 billion annually, including $44 billion for direct medical care and $54 billion for indirect costs associated with disability, work loss, and premature mortality.
- Persons diagnosed with diabetes are at twice the risk of death as those without diabetes.
- Diabetes is the sixth-leading cause of death and the primary cause of blindness, non-traumatic amputations of lower extremities, and kidney failure among adults

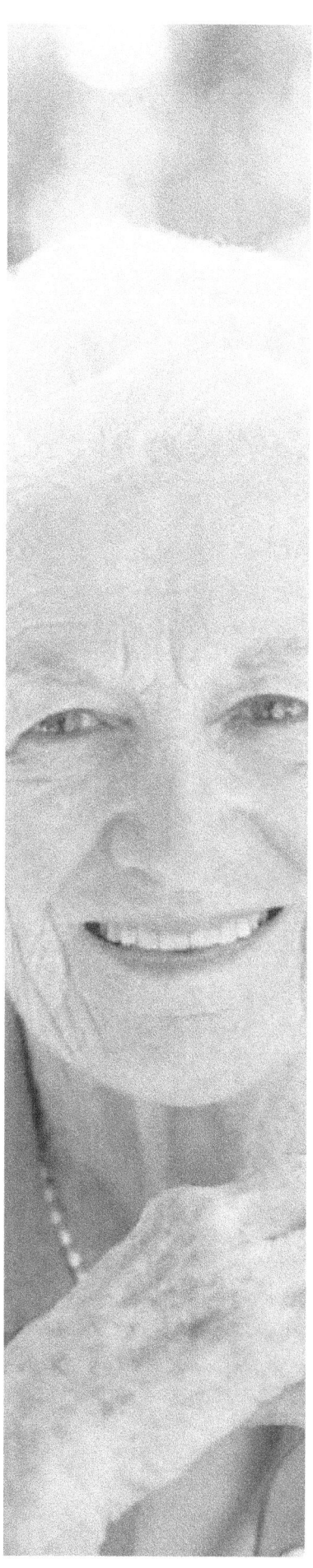

3

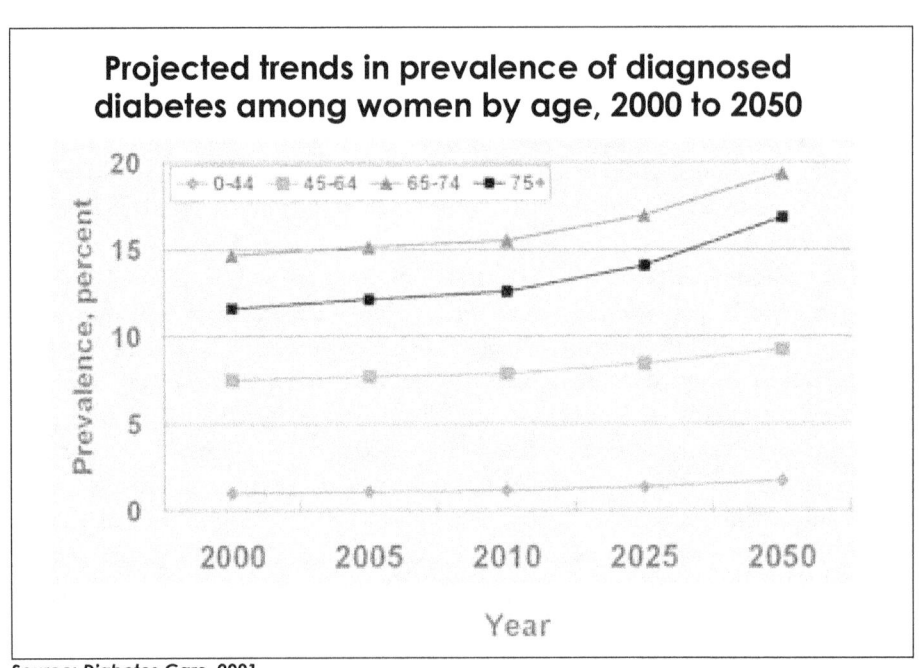

**Projected trends in prevalence of diagnosed diabetes among women by age, 2000 to 2050**

Source: *Diabetes Care*, 2001

### *The Effects of Diabetes on Women Are Unique and Profound*

- More than half (9.1 million) of the cases of diabetes occur among women.
- From 1990 to 2000, the prevalence of diabetes increased almost 50% among women.
- The prevalence of diabetes among women aged 45-55 years was less than 2% in the 1960s, but rose consistently in the 1980s and 1990s. In the early 1990s, the rate was about 6%.
- Women in minority racial and ethnic groups are the hardest hit by type 2 diabetes; the prevalence is about two to four times higher among black, Hispanic, American Indian, and Asian Pacific Islander women than among white women. Because minority populations are expected to grow at a faster rate than the U.S. population as a whole, the number of women in these groups who are diagnosed with diabetes will increase significantly over the coming years.
- Diabetes is a more powerful cause of heart disease among women than men.
- The prognosis of heart disease, the most common complication of diabetes, is more serious among women than men. Among persons with diabetes who have had a heart attack, women have lower survival rates and poorer quality of life than men do.
- Many older women with diabetes live alone and are poor. Poverty is also a major concern for women of childbearing age who have diabetes.

### *Diabetes Affects Women at Various Life Stages Differently*

*The Adolescent Years (10-17 Years)*

- About 61,500 females younger than 20 years old have type 1 diabetes; 92% are white, 4% are black, and 4% are Hispanic or Asian American.
- Type 2 diabetes is now being diagnosed more frequently among youth of all

4

racial and ethnic groups and is more commonly diagnosed among girls than boys.

- The rate of death is nearly five times greater among girls with type 1 diabetes than among the general population of girls aged 10-17 years.
- By age 20 years, 40%-60% of persons with diabetes have retinopathy, or diabetic eye disease. Retinopathy can lead to blindness if untreated. The risk for developing proliferative retinopathy, the most severe form, is higher for girls than boys.
- Eating disorders may be higher among young women with type 1 diabetes than among young women in the general population.

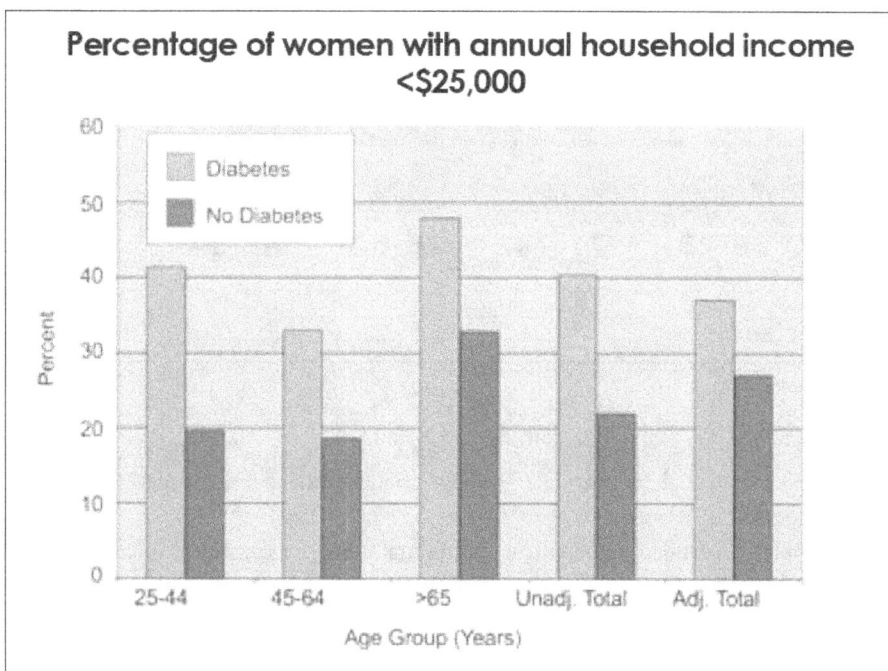

**Percentage of women with annual household income <$25,000**

Adjusted for age, race/ethnicity, marital status, size of household, and employment status.

Source: BRFSS, 2000

*The Reproductive Years (18-44 Years)*

- An estimated 1.85 million women of reproductive age have diabetes; about 500,000 of them do not know they have the disease.
- The death rate for women aged 25-44 years with diabetes is more than three times the rate for those without diabetes.
- Women of minority racial and ethnic groups are about two to four times more likely than non-Hispanic white women to have type 2 diabetes.
- Estimates of the overall prevalence of gestational diabetes in the United States range from 2.5% to 4% of pregnancies that result in live births. Most cases of this type of diabetes result from the body's resistance to the action of insulin and may be precipitated by the increased insulin resistance that normally occurs during pregnancy.
- Gestational diabetes usually ends after the baby is born, but women with

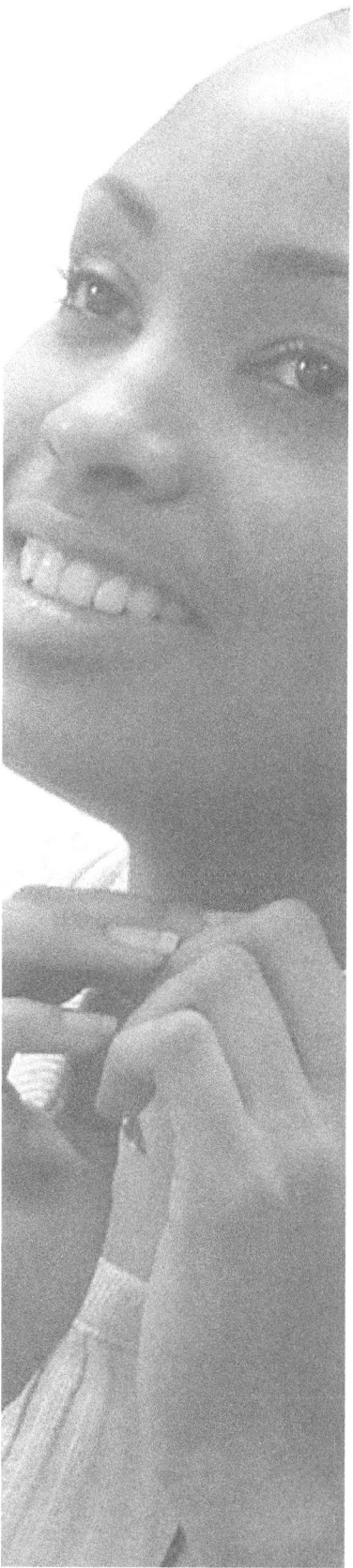

5

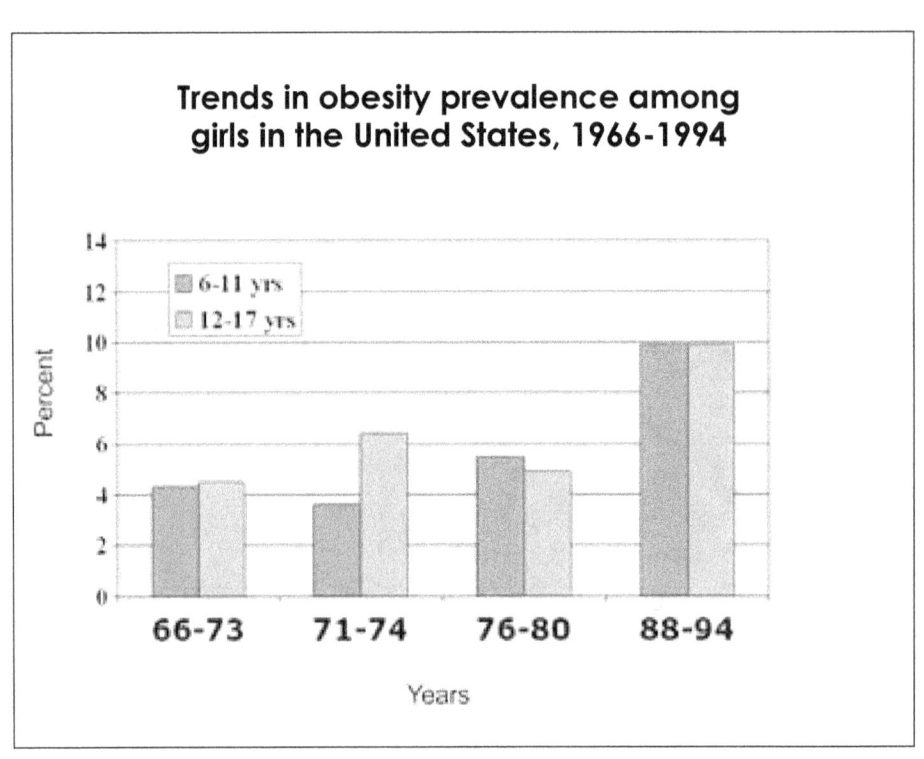

**Trends in obesity prevalence among girls in the United States, 1966-1994**

Source: *Pediatrics*, 1998

gestational diabetes have a 20%-50% chance of developing type 2 diabetes in the next 5-10 years.

- Poorly controlled diabetes during the first trimester can result in congenital malformations and spontaneous abortions, while in the second and third trimesters of pregnancy it can result in excessively large babies, posing a risk to both the mother and child during delivery.
- Children exposed to diabetes in utero have a greater likelihood of becoming obese during childhood and adolescence and of developing type 2 diabetes later in life.

*The Middle Years (45-64 Years)*

- Approximately 1.73 million women aged 45-64 years have diabetes.
- For middle-aged women, type 2 diabetes is at least twice as common among racial and ethnic minority groups as among whites.
- Diabetes is a leading cause of death among middle-aged American women.
- Coronary heart disease is an important cause of illness among middle-aged women with diabetes; rates are three to seven times higher among women 45-64 years old with diabetes than those without diabetes.
- In 2000, at least one in four women aged 45-64 years with diabetes had a low level of formal education, and one in three lived in a low-income household. Women with diabetes were more likely to have a low socioeconomic status regardless of race, ethnicity, or living arrangements (marital status, size of household, and employment status).

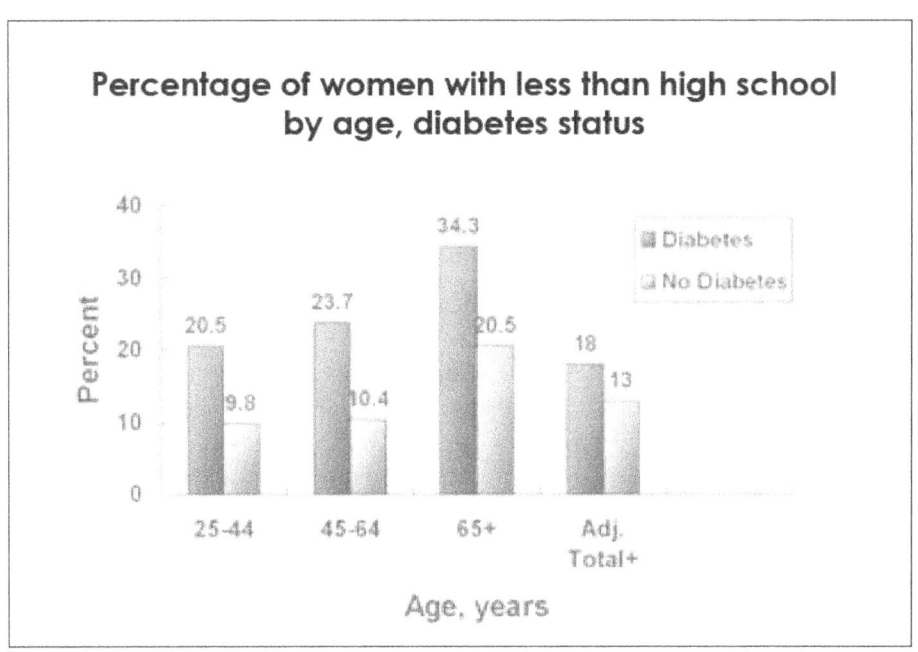

## Percentage of women with less than high school by age, diabetes status

Percent (y-axis, 0 to 40)

- 25-44: Diabetes 20.5, No Diabetes 9.8
- 45-64: Diabetes 23.7, No Diabetes 10.4
- 65+: Diabetes 34.3, No Diabetes 20.5
- Adj. Total+: Diabetes 18, No Diabetes 13

Age, years

Adjusted for age, race/ethnicity, marital status, size of household, and employment status.

Source: BRFSS, 2000

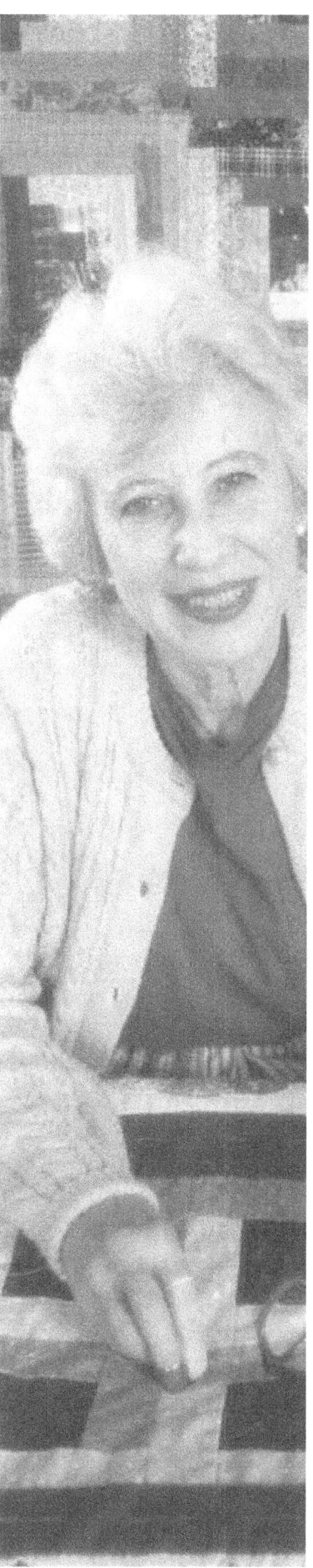

*The Older Years (65 Years and Older)*
- About 4.5 million women aged 60 years and older have diabetes; one quarter of them do not know they have the disease. Most elderly women with diabetes have type 2 diabetes.
- On average, women live longer than men. Because elderly women live longer than men, there are nearly twice as many older women than men. Elderly women with diabetes also outnumber elderly men with diabetes. Diabetes is one of the leading underlying causes of death among women aged 65 years and older.
- Being older and having diabetes accelerate diabetic complications such as heart disease, stroke, kidney disease, and blindness. Elderly women with diabetes are at particularly high risk for heart disease, visual problems, hyperglycemia or hypoglycemia, and depression.

*Factors That Place Women at Risk for Diabetes and Its Complications*
Women face increasing risk of diabetes and its complications because of certain social and economic trends. Increasing numbers of women:
- live in poverty (by age 65, women are twice as likely as men to be poor),
- are employed (women tend to work in small companies that provide fewer benefits and lower pay than larger companies, and often struggle to balance job and family responsibilities),
- are uninsured and lack access to health care (approximately one in seven women lacks health insurance),
- are overweight and do not exercise regularly (about one-third of women aged

7

20 years or older are overweight, and nearly two-thirds do not engage in regular physical activity),

- live alone, particularly as they get older (women live an average of 7 years longer than men; by age 75, women outnumber men by a ratio of 2 to 1), and

- are members of racial and ethnic minority populations (who tend to be diagnosed with type 2 diabetes more often).

### Initiative on Diabetes and Women's Health

As part of a comprehensive effort to improve women's health, the Centers for Disease Control and Prevention (CDC) established the National Public Health Initiative on Diabetes and Women's Health. The initiative has three phases. In **Phase I**, *Diabetes & Women's Health Across the Life Stages: A Public Health Perspective* was prepared. This report, published in 2001, examines the issues that make diabetes a serious public health problem for women; analyzes the epidemiologic, psychosocial, socioeconomic, and environmental dimensions of women and diabetes; and discusses the public health implications. This landmark document explores the impact of diabetes on women's lives by using a framework that defines the issues across various life stages: the adolescent, reproductive, middle, and elderly years. A complete copy is available on CDC's website at http://www.cdc.gov/diabetes/pubs/pdf/women.pdf.

Following Phase I, CDC joined forces with the American Diabetes Association (ADA), the American Public Health Association (APHA), and the Association of State and Territorial Health Officials (ASTHO) to convert the information contained in the 2001 report into a plan of action (**Phase II**). Toward this end, the four cosponsoring agencies formed a task force of selected individuals representing over 40 organizations from the public, private, and voluntary sectors. The task force convened on November 1-2, 2001, in Washington, D.C., to begin to identify needed strategies, policies, surveillance, and research for improving the lives of women diagnosed with or at risk for diabetes. Recommendations that emerged from this meeting were compiled into a draft document, which was circulated to task force members and other experts for review. The result was this *Interim Report: Proposed Recommendations for Action*.

**Phase III** of the initiative will involve preparing and implementing the National Public Health Action Plan on Diabetes and Women's Health. The proposed recommendations contained in the interim report will be expanded during a working summit in August, 2002. At this meeting, invited officials from multidisciplinary agencies (including government, academic, voluntary, business, community-based, and professional organizations) will become more familiar with the proposed recommendations from Phase II, select those of highest priority, identify appropriate strategies for implementation, recommend lead agencies for implementation, and propose time frames for action and results. Attendees will include representatives of many of the organizations on the task force, along with others likely to have a major role in implementation.

## STRATEGIC FRAMEWORK
### Vision and Goals

The ultimate vision of the National Public Health Initiative on Diabetes and Women's Health is to:

- prevent diabetes among women whenever possible,
- promote early diagnosis and appropriate management of diabetes among women across the life stages,
- prevent, delay, or minimize complications from diabetes among women, and
- educate the families and communities of women at risk for diabetes, and provide the support they need to prevent diabetes and its complications.

With this vision as a foundation, the Initiative's specific goals are to work within the framework of *Healthy People 2010* to:

- garner the national attention of policy makers, public health professionals, other advocates for women's issues, researchers, and the general public that diabetes is a prominent public health issue,
- develop consensus among key stakeholders that there is a need to develop priority strategies, policies, and research to improve diabetes and women's health,
- delineate the public health role in diabetes and women's health at national, state, and community levels, and improve the capacity of these public health sectors to fulfill that role,
- unite partners from multiple sectors of society in a coordinated strategy to prevent and manage diabetes among women, and
- empower women to adopt prevention strategies that will improve their overall health and will delay or prevent diabetes and its complications.

### Guiding Principles

The guiding principles underlying the National Public Health Initiative on Diabetes and Women's Health are as follows:

- A public health approach to diabetes among women should be adopted. This approach aims to improve the health and quality of life for all women primarily through prevention and focuses on all factors influencing health status: physical, behavioral, psychological, and socioeconomic.
- **Collaboration** within and between multiple sectors of society is essential for success. These sectors include public and private health care organizations, business and industry, education and environment, communication and media, and policy makers.
- Strategies and policies must fully consider and take into account the unique needs of women in different life stages among all racial, ethnic, religious, and cultural groups.
- Women and grassroots organizations should be fully engaged as active partners in policy decisions and in program planning, implementation, and evaluation. The strong involvement and support of men should be sought as well.
- Leadership of state and community agencies and groups must share accountability for adopting approaches to improve the health status of women.

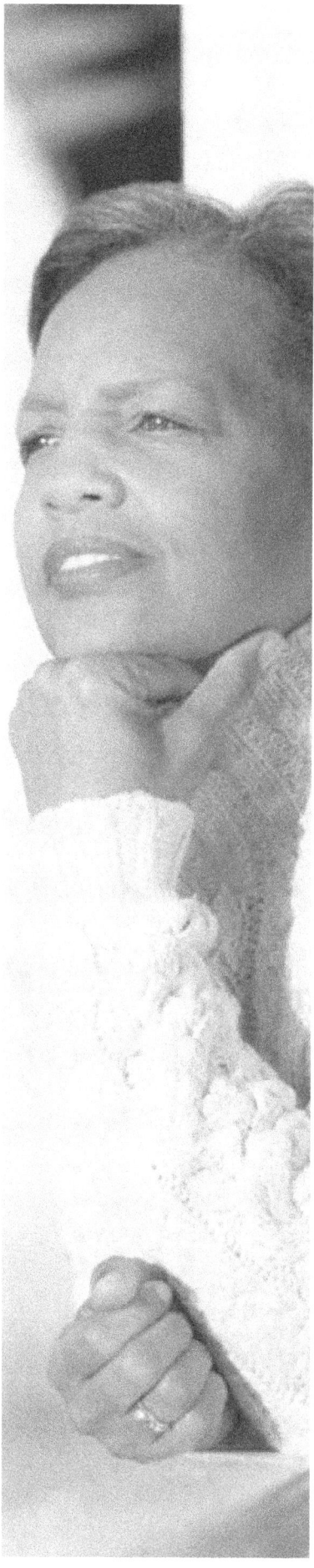

9

- Actions should be based on **sound research** from all relevant scientific fields, and the pursuit of additional research should focus on filling gaps in scientific knowledge. Assessment must guide policy and program development.
- **Measurable outcomes** for programs and policies should be established so that progress and impact can be evaluated and approaches can be modified as needed.
- Strategies and policies must be **sustainable and integrated** over time, not just one-time activities or interventions. New initiatives should build on existing resources, services, and natural links between local, state, and federal agencies and organizations in both the public and private sectors.

## Public Health Prevention Framework

### Levels of Prevention

The recommendations in this report encompass three levels of prevention. **Primary prevention** aims to prevent diabetes from occurring among women. **Secondary prevention** aims to identify diabetes at its earliest stage so that prompt and appropriate management can be initiated. Successful secondary prevention reduces the negative impact of diabetes on a woman's life. The goal of **tertiary prevention** is to reduce or minimize the consequences of diabetes once it has developed. That is, to eliminate, or at least delay and reduce, the onset and severity of complications and disability due to diabetes.

### Life Stages

These recommendations also recognize the unique challenges to prevent diabetes and its complications among women in different life stages. The **adolescent years** (ages 10-17 years) are marked by major biological and psychosocial changes that transform adolescents into adults. Many adolescents with diabetes face life choices that can affect their ability to control the disease. Primary prevention and instituting lifelong healthy behaviors related to physical activity and nutrition are key in this lifestage. The **reproductive years** (ages 18-44 years) represent the life stage in which women experience significant personal growth and responsibility: additional schooling, marriage, career development, and child rearing. Diabetes during pregnancy, regardless of type, puts both a woman and her unborn child at risk for negative health outcomes. For those with few personal resources, diabetes during pregnancy can place them at high risk for negative outcomes and future economic hardship. The **middle years** (ages 45-64 years) are noted by major physiological events such as menopause. This is also a time when other chronic diseases or complications of diabetes most often first appear, along with many other social and psychological changes such as disability, death of a significant other or parent, divorce, and retirement. Because women are increasingly developing diabetes at younger ages, the development of complications will occur earlier as well. The **older years** (ages 65 years and over) are when women with diabetes become even more vulnerable to other chronic illnesses, disability, poverty, and loss of social support systems. The number of women in this age group is growing exponentially as the American population ages.

### Categories of Recommendations

Many of the recommendations for public health action pertain to all women, regardless of life stage; others are life stage-specific. Presented in the following two sections of this report, these recommendations are divided into two categories.

Strategy and policy recommendations address communication and education of families, health care providers, and other professionals who may serve patients; and services and programs to improve the effectiveness of interventions in schools, work sites, health care systems, and other community organizations and settings. Disease Tracking and research recommendations encourage further knowledge of the epidemiologic, socioenvironmental, behavioral, translational, and biomedical factors that influence diabetes and women's health.

While the focus of these recommendations is to improve the health and well-being of women, adopting and implementing many of these recommendations will also benefit men and families.

## STRATEGY AND POLICY RECOMMENDATIONS

Many state and local agencies and organizations, including the diabetes control programs supported in large part by CDC, are engaged in the prevention and control of diabetes. However, significantly large gaps exist in the tools, capacities, and resources of these organizations. To fill these gaps, this section presents recommended strategies and policies of highest priority for action in the next 3-5 years. Recommendations encompass two major areas: Communication and Education and Services and Programs. Included in the area of **communication and education** are recommendations for increasing awareness of diabetes among women, the disease's impact on women's health, effective prevention strategies, and the importance of early diagnosis and management. Strategies and policies target women in each of the life stages, as well as their families, health care providers, and other professionals who may serve them. Recommendations in the area of **services and programs** aim to improve the effectiveness of services at the local, state, and national levels to prevent and manage diabetes among women. They encompass strategies and policies for schools, work sites, health care systems, and other community organizations and settings.

### All Women

Several key strategy and policy recommendations pertain to women of all ages, regardless of their life stage. Some of these recommendations also appear later in this report, in the context of a specific life stage.

- **Strengthen advocacy on behalf of women** with or at risk for diabetes, either by constituting a new organization focused exclusively on the issues related to diabetes and women's health, or by forming a consortium of existing organizations with missions that encompass diabetes, chronic disease, and quality of life for women.
- **Increase awareness among the general public** of the seriousness and preventability of diabetes in women. Using social marketing approaches, educational programs should be designed to appropriately consider age, language, literacy level, culture, race, ethnicity, motivation, and other relevant factors including access to personal, family, and community resources.
- **Expand community-based health promotion** education, activities, and incentives for all ages in a wide variety of settings such as: schools, workplaces, senior centers, churches, civic organizations, and the like. Of particular

11

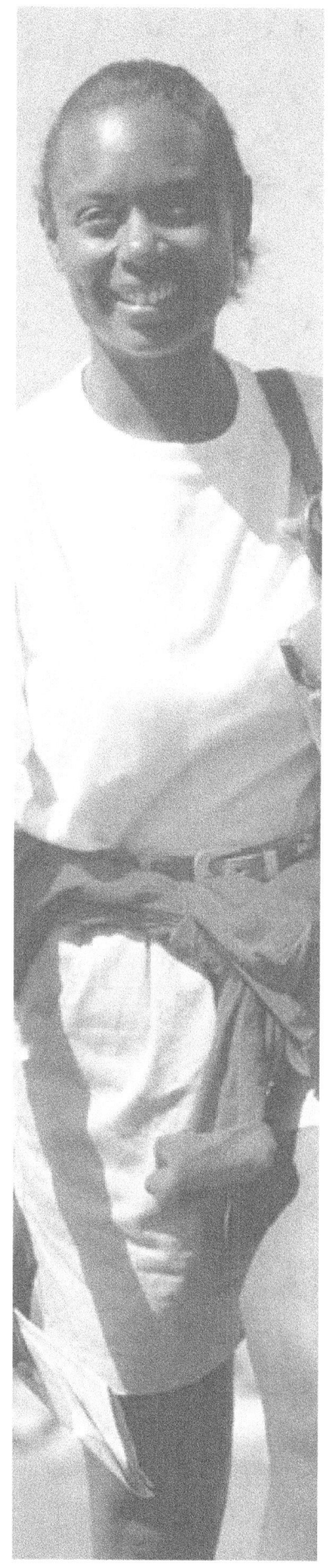

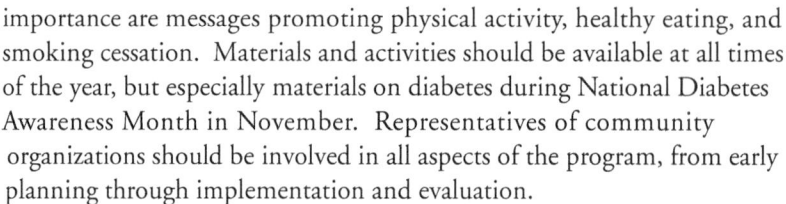

importance are messages promoting physical activity, healthy eating, and smoking cessation. Materials and activities should be available at all times of the year, but especially materials on diabetes during National Diabetes Awareness Month in November. Representatives of community organizations should be involved in all aspects of the program, from early planning through implementation and evaluation.

- **Integrate diabetes messages** and prevention activities within the larger context of chronic disease prevention and health promotion. Health organizations should strive to cooperate, strategize, and plan public health initiatives with organizations in other sectors, such as education, parks and recreation, city planning, and businesses.

- **Enhance community development policies and practices** (including "smart growth" initiatives and empowerment zones) that promote safe environments for physical activity such as: recreational facilities and activities, parks, side-walks, mass transit, well-lit neighborhoods.

- **Increase availability of and access to healthy food choices** for all sectors of the population. This recommendation is particularly important for urban and economically disadvantaged populations.

- **Support policies and programs in schools and workplaces** that respect the health-related needs of their female students and employees, particularly women with or at risk for diabetes, and facilitate prevention and self-management of the disease.

- **Fortify community programs** with:
  - guidelines on education strategies at different levels of funding, including tips for developing multisectoral coalitions, implementing strategies, ways to use available resources most efficiently, discussion of resource allocation issues to aid decision making, and suggestions for accessing extant resources,
  - performance measures for evaluating diabetes activities,
  - dissemination of "best practices" and lessons learned from community programs and in workplace and school settings (for example, physical activity programs, health coverage, healthy cafeteria foods, and support groups),
  - enhanced funding opportunities,
  - simplified processes for securing financial support from federal, state, and local agencies, and
  - technical assistance (such as workshops and mentoring) to help state and local policy makers prepare and submit successful proposals to potential government and private funding sources.

- **Assure access to trained health care providers** who offer quality services to prevent and manage diabetes among women of all ages. Care should be tailored to the woman's specific life stage, race, ethnicity, culture, religion, family and financial situation, motivation, and needs.

- **Expand public and private health insurance packages** to provide adequate coverage for preventive care, including health promotion, health and nutritional education, physical activity, self-management, and screening for complications among women diagnosed with diabetes.

12

## The Adolescent Years (ages 10-17 years)

The primary emphasis of public health action in the adolescent years is to improve the health and preventive practices among all youth, and more particularly among girls already diagnosed with diabetes. To accomplish this goal, several major challenges must be overcome. These challenges include: lack of diabetes education and prevention materials appropriate for adolescent females; inadequate numbers of trained physicians who specialize in caring for this age group; lack of physical education programs in schools; lack of awareness of the need for weight control, healthy diets, and physical activity among adolescents; and a plethora of fast food and other unhealthy eating options.

Opportunities for prevention and hope for the future are influenced by recent school policy changes and better models for physical education and health education curriculum. Successes for other diseases and health problems that might benefit diabetes prevention efforts (such as, no-smoking and Drug Abuse Resistance Education [DARE] campaigns) include: more effective media messages to raise awareness and promote healthy lifestyles; advances in electronic and computer technology as a teaching tool; and the receptivity of adolescents to computer technology.

### Communication and Education
*For Professionals*

- Examine and improve the health professional school curriculum as it relates to preventing diabetes complications among adolescents.
- Strengthen continuing education and training for physicians, nurses, and other health care providers on adolescent weight control, glucose management, eating disorders, and other diabetes prevention and management issues relevant to female adolescents with or at high risk of diabetes.
- Explore establishing a subspecialty of physicians on diabetes care for female adolescents.
- Target dentists to help prevent periodontal disease in adolescents, particularly girls, with type 1 diabetes.

*For Adolescent Females and Their Families*

- Develop family-oriented education materials covering such topics as nutrition, physical activity, and a family's risk of diabetes and other chronic diseases.
- Begin to introduce concepts of reproductive health to adolescents and their families, particularly the relationship between poor contraception and congenital anomalies.
- Structure educational messages to encourage female adolescents with diabetes to engage in regular physical activity and make healthy food choices in the face of the vast fast food market.
- Use teen media outlets, entertainers, and community "champions" (including teen performers with diabetes) to deliver key messages to adolescent females. Search for positive images and role models for girls that, for example, emphasize being "strong" rather than "thin."
- Target gestational diabetes and broader family health messages to pregnant adolescents, urging the teens to, for example, get their glucose level checked.
- Educate recipients of public assistance (such as food stamps and Women,

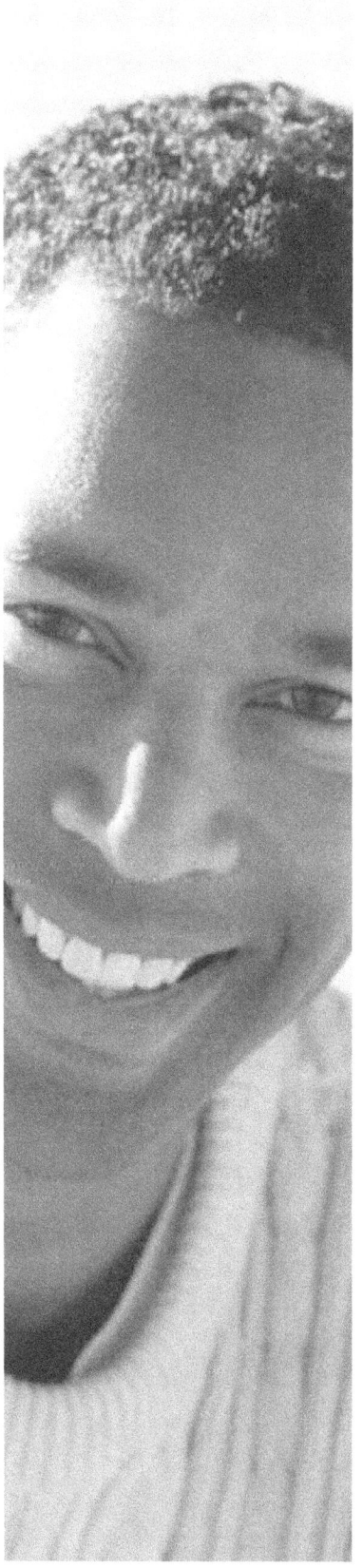

Infants and Children [WIC] program services) on preparing healthy and appetizing meals within a limited budget for families with an adolescent with diabetes.

## Services and Programs

### In Communities

- Create positive, rewarding forums that promote healthy eating and physical activity among adolescent females. Partner with established groups such as Girl Scouts and Girl Power, and use locations where adolescents typically congregate. Consider such programs as "teen summits" (similar to the Black Entertainment Television's Teen Summit program), visits to local cable channel stations, and televised "town hall meetings" on health issues. Involve young girls in the planning and delivery of these programs whenever possible.
- Establish appealing and acceptable alternatives to competitive sports for those adolescent females who would otherwise not engage in any physical activity.
- Expand support groups (at YWCAs, churches, and other grassroots organizations' sites) for adolescent girls with diabetes and their families.

### In Schools

- Integrate health into the school science curriculum and supplement with activities that directly influence adolescents, such as videos and guest speakers with thought-provoking messages that have been shown to change behavior.
- Conduct awareness campaigns to influence parental behavior to prevent and manage diabetes among children. Heighten sensitivity to the challenges of disease management specific to adolescents.
- Urge community and state boards of health and education to allocate more funding for physical activity programs in public schools offered before, during, and after school.
- Develop school policies that limit soda and candy vending machine availability in schools (or support vending machines for healthy snacks and drinks), and promote healthy food choices in cafeterias.
- Advocate for national support of on-site school nurses to aid youth diagnosed with diabetes and other health problems.
- Educate school system administrators and teachers about diabetes and its management so that a "diabetes friendly" environment can be established and medical emergencies avoided or handled appropriately.

### In Work Sites

- Educate employers of adolescents, such as retailers, grocery stores, fast food restaurants, and other restaurants, about the risks for diabetes among adolescents and the need for adequate breaks, healthy food choices, and health insurance.

### In Health Care Systems

- Promote early diagnosis and self-management of diabetes, particularly type 2 diabetes, among health care providers.
- Encourage guidelines that trigger interventions for adolescents at risk of

developing type 2 diabetes. Risk factors include low waist-to-hip ratio and an apple-shaped body type.
- Define a healthy weight loss regimen for overweight adolescents, focusing on the influences of family and school.
- Encourage health insurance companies to cover health and nutrition education for adolescents (for example, management of obesity and eating disorders).
- Develop population-specific messages, materials, and programs for health insurance or pharmaceutical companies to use for diabetes education and self-management among adolescents.
- Collaborate with diabetes control programs in state health departments to develop prevention efforts among adolescents.

## The Reproductive Years (ages 18-44 years)

One of the major barriers to self-care facing women in their reproductive years is balancing the demands of marriage and other relationships, work, child care, household chores and hobbies. The result is limited time for physical activity, healthy eating patterns, and attending to the woman's own health care needs. In addition, physical activity is further restricted during pregnancy and early postpartum. Mothers may not lose the weight gained during pregnancy and thus put themselves at greater risk of obesity and of developing diabetes in later pregnancies or later in life. Cultural differences influencing these behaviors are also important to understand. Conflicting health messages from a multitude of sources addressing chronic disease prevention is another barrier to self-care.

Strategies for countering these barriers include tailoring messages to reproductive-aged women, capitalizing on the intergenerational aspects of gestational diabetes, and including men and families as supportive partners. Prenatal and other reproductive health services represent important vehicles for identifying and instituting preventive care for women at high risk for diabetes.

*Communication and Education*
*For Professionals*
- Establish a clearinghouse of programs and materials for women of reproductive age, and disseminate best practices and lessons learned from community programs (such as the National Kidney Foundation's *Healthy Hair Beauty Salon Project* in Michigan) and workplace, clinic, and other settings (for example, exercise programs, health coverage, healthy cafeteria foods, and support groups).
- For health care providers, expand education in diabetes prevention and management, emphasizing such specialties as family planning, obstetrics, gynecology, general practice, family practice, midwifery, and social services (for example, providers in WIC or the Expanded Food and Nutrition Education Program [EFNEP]).
- Encourage makers of drugs and instruments for diabetes management (such as insulin, oral agents, acarbose, and glucose meters) to include a public message in the package encouraging good diabetes control.
- Urge pharmacies to provide information for patients.

15

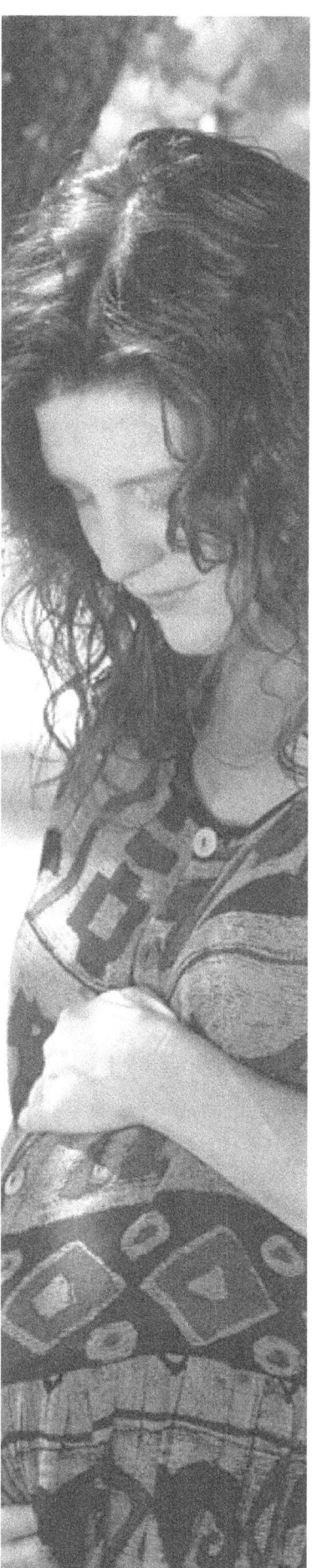

*For Women and Their Families*
- Include lifestyle counseling and education strategies for women with and without diabetes in preconception, prenatal, and postpartum care (including women with or at risk of gestational diabetes). Address contraception and pregnancy planning.
- Emphasize to women, health care providers, and health insurers the importance of appropriate follow-up diagnostic and preventive care after delivery for women with gestational diabetes and other risk factors for type 2 diabetes.
- Increase diabetes awareness programs and materials in workplaces and other settings, such as drug stores, health clinics, the media, community recreational centers, school newsletters, and church bulletins.
- Review educational materials produced by organizations serving women of reproductive age (such as March of Dimes; Healthy Mothers, Healthy Babies Coalition; and Maternal and Child Health Bureau) to ensure inclusion of appropriate, current, and consistent information regarding diabetes and related risks (for example, obesity, poor diet, and physical inactivity). Materials should also be culturally and linguistically appropriate.
- Educate women with diabetes and prior gestational diabetes about the risk to their offspring for developing diabetes. Establish a follow-up program to test these children.

## Services and Programs

*In Communities*
- Provide opportunities to support and sustain lifestyle changes among women of reproductive age, including
  - assessment and counseling within the framework of existing programs and services, and linking to other available resources,
  - peer and other social support programs geared toward women for exercise, healthy eating, and diabetes self-management, and
  - assessment of family and community barriers specific to this age group, such as lack of access to affordable child care.
- Evaluate existing community programs to maximize opportunities for prevention activities, improved quality, and increased access to health care among women in their reproductive years.
- Adapt existing resources to the needs of reproductive-aged women, and ensure appropriate support services such as child care to enable time for physical activity.

*In Schools*
- Use school sites as a way to reach women in their reproductive years, such as students, mothers of students, and female teachers, with prevention and management messages.
- Influence policies of colleges and universities to require a minimum number of hours of physical education and to include healthy food options in cafeteria food plans.
- Encourage colleges and universities to promote exercise, dance, and other physical activities for females.

- Promote partnerships between health care providers and workplaces, and encourage employers and employees to discuss needed diabetes benefits in the health package offered.
- Promote workplace policies that positively affect the health of women of reproductive age, such as flextime for exercise on lunch hours, shower facilities, health club memberships, and support for insulin breaks.
- Promote purchasing cooperatives among small businesses to enable progressive health insurance packages.

*In Health Care Systems*
- Develop a chronic disease prevention policy for reproductive-aged women, and enhance cooperation among state and community chronic disease programs to support common prevention strategies (for example, exercise, nutrition, and smoking cessation).
- Ensure that all women who have had or are at risk for gestational diabetes are identified, treated, and followed up regularly over time in traditional and nontraditional settings (for example, WIC, mobile outreach services, family planning clinics, Indian Health Service clinics, and community health centers).
- Assure postpartum follow-up to assess risk factors, conduct diagnostic testing for diabetes with other routine tests, and recommend preventive strategies. Use existing programs such as WIC and the State Children's Health Insurance Program to reach at-risk women to promote preventive activities, and provide tools that health care providers can incorporate into routine care. Expand activities like "Project Fresh" in WIC programs to encourage fresh fruit and vegetable consumption.
- Promote expansion of routine physical examinations of reproductive-aged women to include assessments of physical activity, diet, hip and waist measurements, and body mass index in addition to standard weight and blood pressure measurements. Glucose screening should also be performed if the woman is significantly overweight and has one or more risk factors for diabetes.
- Review existing standards of care for women of childbearing age to determine if the guidelines are comprehensive and whether they have been implemented (for example, those sponsored by the American College of Obstetrics and Gynecology, the American Diabetes Association, the U.S. Preventive Health Services Task Force, and WIC). In addition, the standards and guidelines should be updated as appropriate.
- Modify current policies regarding weight gain during pregnancy to promote appropriate, rather than excessive, weight gain regardless of age or ethnicity.
- Promote comprehensive health care coverage that includes diabetes prevention and management for women of reproductive age.

## The Middle Years (ages 45-64 years)

During this life stage, some of the major barriers to preventing diabetes and its complications are similar to those in the reproductive years. Prevention takes a

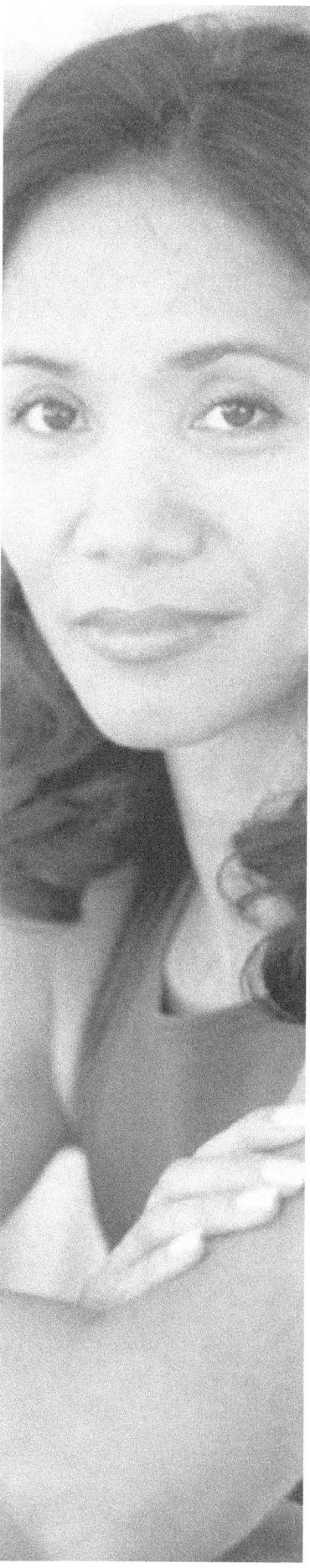

backseat to treatment, particularly for acute health issues. A transition in health care providers occurs, from gynecologists to family practitioners, internists, or specialists. Women may have even less time to focus on their own needs as they begin to care for their children and also for their own parents.

However, this role as the primary decision maker, sandwiched between two generations, affords a rare opportunity. The woman's sphere of influence is broader and deeper than at any other time in her life; she has the chance to be a role model for female relatives and friends. Middle age is also the time when women are most active in civic and religious organizations, offering an ideal site for delivery of prevention messages, interventions, and support.

### Communication and Education
*For Professionals*
- Increase training opportunities for health care professionals to learn how to effectively prevent and manage diabetes in middle-aged women. Consider such mechanisms as continuing education units, web-based training, CD-ROMs, and partnerships with pharmaceutical companies.
- Develop and disseminate a list of successful programs ("best practices") that promote the incorporation of physical activity and healthy eating into the daily routines of women who are employed, raising children, or both.
- Encourage providers to explore the use of both traditional and alternative medicine for preventing and treating diabetes among women in their middle years.

*For Women and Their Families*
- Emphasize physical activities and healthy eating habits appropriate for the middle years, and focus on incorporating them into the daily routines of work and family. Stress that prevention of weight gain, not just weight loss, can prevent diabetes onset.
- Promote self-management among middle-aged women with diabetes, and provide support and education for self-care.
- Develop champions for diabetes among middle-aged women, and use them to deliver messages about the positive benefits of physical activity and healthy eating.

### Services and Programs
*In Communities*
- Encourage policy makers to focus on priorities for women in their middle years:
    - chronic disease in general, and diabetes in particular,
    - modifiable risk factors, such as age-appropriate physical activity within daily life, diet, and smoking,
    - support needs,
    - focus on family and quality of life, and
    - preparation for menopause and retirement.
- Establish community support groups similar to Alcoholics Anonymous (AA) and Weight Watchers designed primarily for middle-aged women with diabetes.

18

- Use pharmacies and other nontraditional sites (such as beauty salons) to reach middle-aged women diagnosed with or at risk of diabetes.

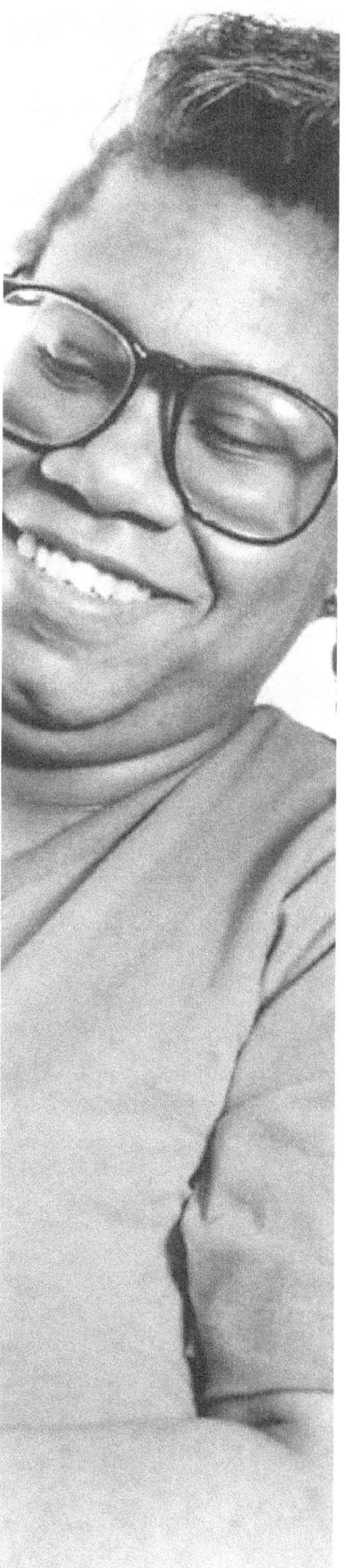

*In Work Sites*
- Promote work site policies that encourage and support physical activity and healthy eating. Highlight diabetes prevention and education.
- Consider using work sites for training and support groups on caregiving.
- Establish "health days" or release days for employees on which they can schedule diagnostic testing for diabetes and other routine medical tests on-site or off-site.

*In Health Care Systems*
- Develop "best practices" for prevention and treatment of diabetes among women in their middle years.
- Work with health insurers and policy makers to expand reimbursement policies to include prevention services for women throughout their life span.
- Integrate diagnostic testing for diabetes with routine tests for other chronic diseases, such as mammograms, Pap smears, and colonoscopies).

## The Older Years (ages 65 and older)

Health insurance barriers are compounded in the older years, with the transition from employer-based coverage to Medicare and other private or public health insurance carriers. The elderly also frequently experience isolation, depression, and lack of social support from their families and communities. Prescription drug coverage is an issue, as is the fragmentation of health care services. Financial resources may be limited, particularly for those relying on Social Security and fixed incomes. In addition, the number of elderly persons from racial and ethnic minority populations who have limited English proficiency is increasing dramatically, with no comparable increase in the availability of culturally and linguistically appropriate health care services.

Opportunities for prevention lie in the frequency of health care visits among the elderly for diabetes and comorbidities. Although the actual face-to-face time with health care providers is limited, that time can be optimally used for meaningful education and motivational messages. Community, civic, and religious organizations can also play key roles in promoting behaviors that improve health and quality of life.

### Communication and Education
*For Professionals*
- Encourage health care providers to become aware of and inform their elderly patients about relevant community services.
- Train nurses, other clinic staff, and lay educators on key messages for older women with or at risk of diabetes (for example, about the need for foot screening).
- Incorporate training on cultural competence into the curriculum of all health care professions, particularly for providers who interact with older women.
- Train housing managers, community health workers, and senior center workers on how to recognize signs of depression and how to respond appropriately to those signs.

*For Women and Their Families*
- Promote self-management and education through advocacy and training for the elderly and their health care providers and through expanded availability of quality programs.
- Design a media campaign targeted to elderly women, with a diabetes champion (a celebrity or community leader) as spokesperson.
- Use mainstream media that will reach older women, such as the popular magazines Good Housekeeping, Ladies' Home Journal, and Readers Digest and the American Association of Retired Persons (AARP) newsletters.
- Educate seniors on lifestyle changes that prevent and treat diabetes, including physical activity, healthy eating, and relieving depression. Emphasize all the diseases that typically have onset in later life and their relationships (for example, between heart disease and diabetes).

### Services and Programs
*In Communities*
- Build community coalitions that involve the elderly and address their unique needs.
- Identify key places and organizations to reach the elderly (such as libraries, grocery stores, senior centers, Lions Clubs, churches, Area Agencies on Aging and other non-traditional, non-health care organizations) and involve them in program planning and implementation.
- Expand intergenerational programs and activities.
- Partner with local and state commissions on aging to provide transportation for the elderly (such as "Call a Bus"), while also expanding programs that serve the elderly in their homes and congregate living sites to avoid transportation and other motivational issues.

*In Health Care Systems*
- Ensure affordable, accessible, and appropriate care for older women by expanding preventive services, increasing public awareness of diabetes and its burden, and facilitating greater community involvement.
- Increase the priority of federal, state, and local funding for
  - diabetes training for elderly patients and their health care providers,
  - prescription drugs and health insurance coverage, and
  - grassroots and community programs.

## DISEASE TRACKING AND RESEARCH RECOMMENDATIONS

This section highlights priorities for disease tracking and research to further knowledge about the impact of diabetes on women's health. Recommendations are divided into five categories: disease tracking, epidemiologic research, socioenvironmental and behavioral research, translational research, and biomedical research.

**Disease tracking** covers the ongoing and systematic collection, analysis, interpretation, and dissemination of data to understand the nature and extent of diabetes and its complications among women, including changes over time in incidence, prevalence, and risk factors.

**Epidemiologic research questions** address population-based studies to better identify and understand the distribution of diabetes and its risk factors among women.

**Socioenvironmental and behavioral research questions** explore the identification and analysis of social, behavioral, economic, and political factors influencing diabetes and its complications among women.

**Translational research questions** address studies that aim to convert findings from other types of research into practical programs, policies, techniques, and materials for real-world settings.

**Biomedical research questions** involve basic science and clinical research aimed at characterizing the mechanisms and risk factors that influence diabetes and its complications among women. This document emphasizes prevention and public health, but advances in relevant clinical and basic science research could enhance the effectiveness of public health programs and policies.

Recommendations for disease tracking and research questions that pertain to all women are presented first, followed by additional research topics that are pertinent to each life stage.

## All Women
### *Disease Tracking*

To enhance disease tracking of diabetes among women and its impact on their health, the following actions are recommended:

- Define and monitor the geographic distribution of diabetes among females.
- Expand population-based disease tracking to monitor and understand intra-group variations in disease distribution and the factors (such as cultural, racial, ethnic, geographic, demographic, socioeconomic, and genetic) that influence risks for diabetes and complications.
- Establish routine disease tracking of the quality of care for women of childbearing age (for example, the Pregnancy Risk Assessment Monitoring System [PRAMS] for women who have had a recent live birth) and women in later years.
- Routinely collect and analyze disease tracking data by life stage.
- Design disease tracking systems to track and assess where and from whom women are receiving health care.

### *Epidemiologic Research Questions*

- What valid indicators can be used to measure intragroup variations (such as cultural, demographic, socioeconomic, and genetic factors) in disease distribution that influence the risk for diabetes and its complications?
- How do changes in diet, physical activity, psychosocial stress, and work conditions affect the onset of diabetes, particularly for immigrant and disadvantaged populations?

### *Socioenvironmental and Behavioral Research Questions*

- What are some of the psychosocial factors and measures that facilitate (or hinder) successful completion of interventions designed to promote diabetes self-management?
- What are women's perceptions of health care providers' recommendations?
  - To what extent are the recommendations of health care providers

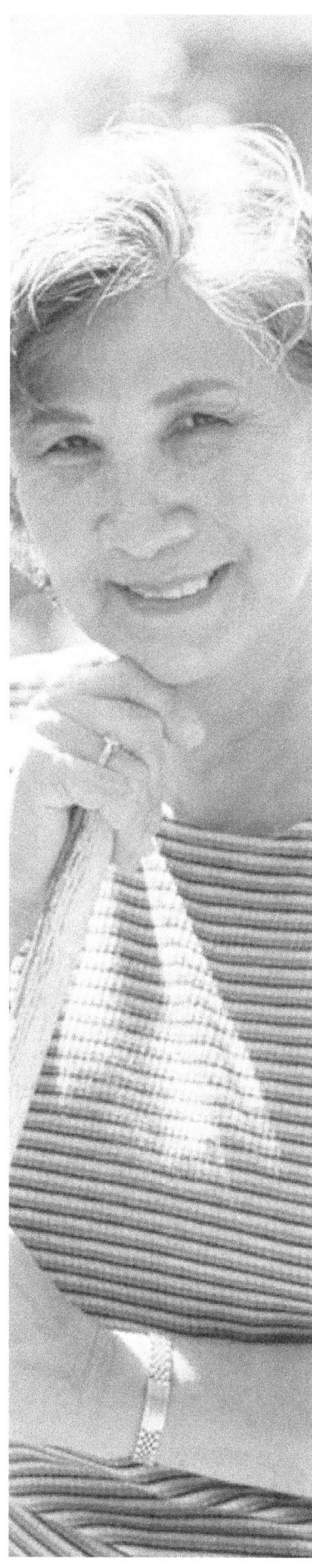

being followed after patients leave the office?
- Do health care professionals clearly explain recommendations and instructions for care so that patients can comprehend them?
- What barriers do women face in trying to follow the recommendations?
• What are the care-seeking behaviors of the uninsured and the working poor?
• How does physical activity change over the life span, and how does this influence the risk for diabetes?
• What is the effect of depression on the lives of women living with diabetes, including their ability to self-manage, obtain adequate health care, and control their risk for diabetes complications?
• How can interventions with immigrant populations encourage physical activity and positive dietary patterns after they move to urban or other new settings?
• What are the best practices for diabetes self-management, use of computerized learning programs, and support groups?
• What is the effect of family structure, income, education, and community factors on diabetes risk, prevention, and care?
• What is the role of social isolation in accelerating risk factors that lead to diabetes and its complications, and at which life stages is it most critical?
• What influence do culturally relevant or health-relevant aspects of religious practice have on health?

## Translational Research Questions
### In Health Communications and Program Design
• What are the knowledge level, attitudes, and perceptions of diabetes risk among health care providers, patients, and the general population, and how do these vary by age, race, ethnicity, and culture?
• What are the community's perceptions of appropriate risk reduction strategies (including programs, resources, and priorities), and to what extent does community-wide "buy-in" exist for application of these strategies?
• How do the history and traditional beliefs of a racial, ethnic, or cultural groups affect health messages and intervention design and delivery about diabetes and its risk factors?
• How can healthy uninsured and underinsured persons be reached, and what messages do they need to hear about diabetes prevention?
• How can women who do not believe in allopathic medicine be reached?
• How can the media be used effectively to reach and mobilize various communities and populations?
- What makes a media message persuasive enough to change behavior?
- Do these elements differ by racial, ethnic, cultural, educational, and religious groups?
• What diabetes education literature is available for women of different ages or life stages, in different languages, and for low-literacy populations?
- What is the quality of that literature?
- Does it cover all aspects of diabetes?
- What adaptations to existing diabetes prevention program materials and methods are needed to be effective for pregnant, postpartum, and nonpregnant women?

- How do women with diabetes rank health issues with regard to primary, secondary, and tertiary care?
    - Do they have different concerns at different life stages or levels of care?
    - What would encourage them to respond differently to these levels?
    - How, where, and from whom do women prefer to receive health information for primary, secondary, and tertiary levels of prevention?
- How can other organizations and programs be convinced to incorporate diabetes messages?
- What are effective ways to encourage women to participate in preventive behaviors?
- What strategies will effectively maintain or increase physical activity and healthy eating at critical times in a woman's life, such as transition to adolescence, pregnancy, or postpartum?
- What are the characteristics of diabetes-related prevention and intervention services that contribute to effective recruitment, retention, and achievement of stated aims for women at different life stages?
- What is the most effective way to identify leadership and empower specific groups of women to promote disease prevention and management?
- How can traditional public health organizations and programs best partner with those outside of public health to benefit women with diabetes?

*In Health Service Delivery*
- How do women define an effective source of diabetes services, and what do women with diabetes look for and want in health services?
- What models of effective diabetes-related preventive care services exist or can be tested?
- What diabetes education classes or medical nutrition therapy classes are available and paid for by health insurance plans?
- What tests and information are various types of health care providers including in their standard examinations and counseling sessions (particularly in settings that serve large numbers of minority patients? Are mutually agreed upon goals established?
- Do health care providers follow accepted guidelines for prevention and management of diabetes?
    - Are there differences in care for different population groups?
    - Are there differences between types of health care providers?
- What strategies can best be used to deliver prevention messages and interventions to patients who present in emergency rooms, and are there opportunities to reach women through other health care professions or venues (such as pharmacies)?
- What are the effects on diabetes care of moving from one health care professional to another as treatment and age demands (for example, from pediatricians to gynecologists or from general practitioners to ophthalmologists), and what are effective strategies for maintaining continuity of care?
- What is the relationship between diagnosis, treatment, and postpartum follow-up of gestational diabetes and the risk for subsequent gestational

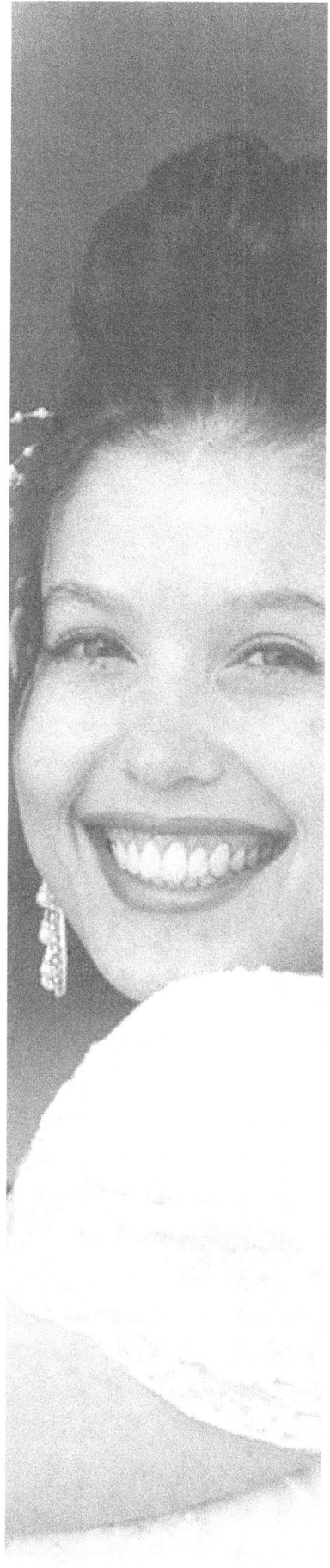

23

diabetes, polycystic ovary syndrome, and type 2 diabetes?
- What strategies best improve communication between health care professionals and women of different cultures, races, ethnicities, ages, and so on?
- Do uninsured and underinsured women, including the working poor, access diabetes care?
  - If so, how?
  - What is the best way to provide services to these women?
- How can employers and health insurers be motivated to include essential elements in their diabetes benefit packages?
- What standardized diagnostic testing protocol (for example, time of day and meals prior to testing) will allow valid comparisons within and between various demographic groups?
- How can the team approach to diabetes care be implemented?

*In Health Economics*
- What is the lifetime cost of health care (including clinical system cost, patient cost, support systems cost, supplies, and equipment) for a woman diagnosed with diabetes at various life stages?
- What are the direct and indirect costs of undiagnosed and untreated diabetes during pregnancy for the mother and her baby?
- What are the costs associated with long-term diabetes prevention programs, such as regular physical activity and healthful eating?
- What are the societal costs of diabetes among women in terms of lost productivity, lost time at work, disability, social assistance, and premature death?
- What are the most cost-effective interventions, both traditional and nontraditional?
- How do changes in cost or health insurance coverage affect outcomes?

*Biomedical Research Questions*
- What is the natural history of the development of diabetes in women?
- What are the most critical periods (fetal, perinatal, childhood, adolescence) for an intervention to have maximum affect on long-term outcomes?
- How can we advocate that biomedical research involve more women? How can we extrapolate biomedical research findings from men to women?

## The Adolescent Years (ages 10-17 years)

Many of the research questions listed in the previous section pertain to adolescents. This section highlights additional questions unique to the life stage that encompasses females aged 10-17 years.

*Epidemiologic Research Questions*
- Does the level of physical activity change during the adolescent years?
  - If so, how and why?
  - How does this affect the risk for diabetes?
- How nutritious are school lunches, and what types of snacks and drinks are offered in school vending machines?

- What is the content and quality of physical education classes and curricula?
- What percentage of adolescents participate in organized sports or other physical activity, and with what health benefits?

## Socioenvironmental and Behavioral Research Questions
- What are the effects of peer pressure and other psychosocial factors on eating habits and participation in physical activity during adolescence, and how do they vary by culture, race, ethnicity, or income?
- What is the role of school systems in encouraging environments that enhance diabetes prevention opportunities (for example, increasing diabetes awareness and encouraging physical activity and healthy eating)? Are dietary standards and physical education standards followed?
- What impact have new school, health care, and other social policies over the past decade had on the incidence of diabetes among adolescent females?
- Are female adolescents who work outside the home at more or less risk of developing obesity or diabetes? If so, why?

## Translational Research Questions
### In Health Communications and Program Design
- Who will adolescent females talk to about personal and sensitive health issues?
- What is the impact of advertising on adolescent females' food choices and eating habits and on their participation in physical activity?
- What are adolescent females' perceptions and knowledge about healthy eating and physical activity, and what are the consequences of these perceptions and knowledge?
- Where do adolescent females get diabetes information that they consider important and credible, and what are effective ways to communicate this information to them?
- How can food practices be altered, such as fast food choices, school vending machine selections, and foods served at sporting events and movies?

### In Health Service Delivery
- What is the pediatrician's role in preventing, diagnosing, referring, treating, and following adolescent females with gestational diabetes and polycystic ovary syndrome?
- How well do health care providers distinguish type 1 diabetes and type 2 diabetes developed during adolescence?
- What is the role of school nurses in preventing, identifying, treating, and referring students with diabetes?
- What is the extent of health care professionals' knowledge of the risk factors, diagnosis, and treatment of type 2 diabetes in children?

### In Health Economics
- What are the costs of type 2 diabetes prevention in youth?

## Biomedical Research Questions
- What is the most effective use of insulin versus oral agents among adolescents?

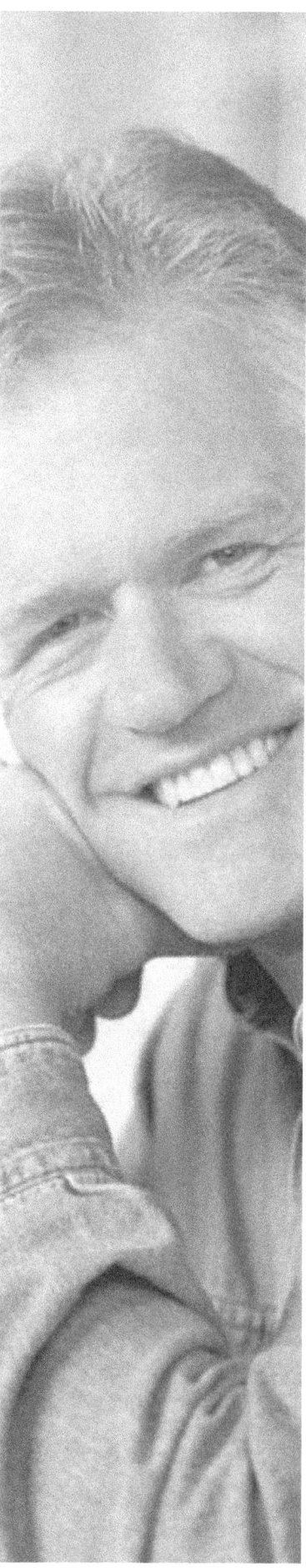

**The Reproductive Years (ages 18-44 years)**

Specific research questions for the life stage covering ages 18-44 years are itemized below.

*Socioenvironmental and Behavioral Research Questions*
- What are the family and community support systems for reproductive-aged women with diabetes, and how can their development be encouraged?
- What are the determinants of women's behavioral of patterns and attitudes regarding physical activity during the reproductive years? How can it be made more socially acceptable to include physical activity and healthy eating as normal parts of everyday life during the reproductive years?
- What is the impact of depression and eating disorders on the lives of reproductive-aged women with diabetes, including their ability to self-manage, obtain adequate health care, and control their risk for diabetes complications?

*Translational Research Questions*
*In Health Communications and Program Design*
- What are the beliefs of health care providers and patients about gestational diabetes, its seriousness, and its consequences, and what is the impact of these beliefs on content and quality of care?
- How can the future risk for developing diabetes be communicated to women diagnosed with gestational diabetes?

*In Health Service Delivery*
- What is the pattern of health care use for reproductive-aged women with diabetes, and how does this pattern vary with socioeconomic status?
- What are the best methods for diagnosing and treating women who may not use reproductive health services?
- Are current standards of prenatal and postpartum diagnosis and follow-up care being followed?
    - At what proportions and with what quality?
    - Which groups of women are most likely to receive inadequate follow-up care?
- What is the extent of postpartum follow-up of women with gestational diabetes and women at high risk of developing diabetes?
- How can existing opportunities or new opportunities be used to identify high-risk women for early intervention and prevention activities (for example, clinics for family planning, prenatal care, postpartum care, or WIC)?
- What is the pediatrician's role in following up with women who have been diagnosed with gestational diabetes?
- What models exist for effective delivery of health care for reproductive-aged women in terms of diabetes prevention and management?

*Biomedical Research Questions*
- Among women of reproductive age, to what extent is depression an indicator or potential risk factor for developing diabetes, eating disorders, or other conditions?
- What effects do changes in weight, diet, and physical activity during and

26

after pregnancy have on the risk of developing gestational diabetes and type 2 diabetes?
- Can early behavioral intervention reduce the risk of gestational diabetes?
- Can effective control of gestational diabetes reduce the woman's risk of subsequent type 2 diabetes?
- What is the interaction between contraception choice and the risk of developing diabetes?

## The Middle Years (ages 45-64 years)

Additional recommendations for research regarding women in the middle years (ages 45-64 years) are listed below.

### Socioenvironmental and Behavioral Research Questions
- What types of health care professionals and health care services do women in middle age seek?
- What is the role of spirituality and natural medicine in maintaining and improving health among middle-aged women with diabetes?
- To what extent does the caretaker role for elderly parents, children, and families interfere with a woman's ability to provide self-care or seek health care services for herself?

### Translational Research Questions
#### In Health Communications and Program Design
- How, where, and from whom do women in middle age prefer to receive health information for primary, secondary, and tertiary levels of care?
- What diabetes education literature and interventions are available for women in their middle years, and how effective are they for different literacy levels, languages, cultures, religions, races, and ethnicities?
- What interventions for diabetes in the middle years will best affect long-term outcomes and improved quality of life?
- How should the delivery of prevention services to middle-aged women with diabetes be designed?

#### In Health Economics
- What affects do diabetes self-management policies have on small and large businesses?

### Biomedical Research Questions
- How can middle-aged women with diabetes and comorbidities be supported and their conditions managed?

## The Older Years (ages 65 and older)

Research questions pertinent to women aged 65 years and older are as follows:

### Socioenvironmental and Behavioral Research Questions
- Are there differences in methods used to alter behaviors related to diet and physical activity later in life than at other life stages?

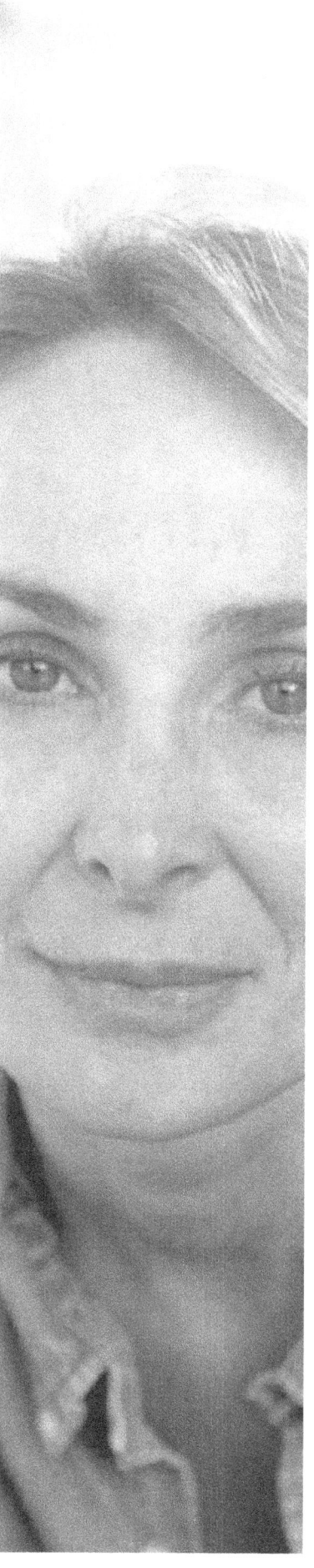

- How are aging networks and other community coalitions being used to reach the elderly with diabetes education, and how effective are they?
- How can peer volunteers and other strategies be best used to support families?
- Are there grassroots organizations, such as churches and beauty shops, which provide ongoing support groups for older women with diabetes?
  - How can additional grassroots organizations be encouraged to get involved?
  - What are other sources of support in the community for older women with diabetes?
- To what extent does caring for a frail, elderly spouse interfere with a woman's ability to provide self-care or seek health care services for herself?

## Translational Research Questions

### In Health Communications and Program Design

- What are the most effective methods for educating the elderly about medical nutrition therapy, detection, comorbidities, and the importance of regular physical activity?
- Are easy-to-read, understandable publications available to help elderly women comprehend how a new diet and physical activity regimen will help control their diabetes?

### In Health Service Delivery

- How can patients' time with a health care worker be maximized to better support the patient in incorporating diabetes management into their lifestyle?
- What are health care providers' perceptions of caring for elderly women with diabetes, and how do these perceptions influence the quality of care and services provided?
- What are the use, compliance, participation, and outcome rates of available health care programs and services for older women?
- How can health care provisions such as prescription drug coverage be ensured for the Medicare population that is underinsured?
- How can the quality of care for the elderly be improved through affordable health insurance, better access to health care, or education for health care providers?

## Biomedical Research Questions

- What is the connection between depression, physical activity, healthy eating, interpersonal relationships, and diabetes in the older years?
- To what extent does multiple prescription drug use in the elderly years interfere with diabetes self-management?
- How is physical activity limited by arthritis, the risk of falls, general frailty, and osteoporosis?

# APPENDIX A:
# TASK FORCE MEMBERS

**Frances Ashe-Goins, RN, MPH**
Director, Policy and Program Development
DHHS/Office on Women's Health
200 Independence Avenue, SW, Room 712E
Washington, DC 20201
Phone: 202-690-7650
Fax: 202-401-4005
E-mailFAshe-Goins@osophs.dhhs.gov

**J. Zoe Beckerman, MPH**
Senior Policy Analyst
Henry J. Kaiser Family Foundation
1450 G Street NW, Suite 250
Washington, DC 20005
Phone: 202-347-5270 ext 126
Fax : 202-347-5274
E-mail: ZBeckerman@kff.org

**Gloria Beckles, MD, MSc**
Medical Epidemiologist, CDC/DDT
4770 Buford Highway, K-10
Atlanta, GA 30341
Phone: 770-488-1272
Fax: 770-488-5966
E-mail: GBeckles@cdc.gov

**Angela Bland, MPH**
Office Automation Clerk, CDC/NCCDPHP/
Office of Communications
4770 Buford Highway, K-40
Atlanta, GA 30341
Phone: 770-488-6419
Fax: 770-488-5962
E-mail: ABland@cdc.gov

**Betty S. Burrier**
Health Insurance Specialist
Centers for Medicare and Medicaid Services
7500 Security Boulevard, MS S1-15-03
Baltimore, MD 21797
Phone: 410-786-4649
Fax: 410-786-8004
E-mail: BBurrier1@cms.hhs.gov

**Ann Constance, RD, MA, CDE**
Past Chair, Public Health Speciality Practice
Group, American Association of Diabetes
Educators, Director, U.P. Diabetes Outreach
Network
102 W. Washington, Suite 232
Marguette Sawyer, MI 49855
Phone: 906-228-9203
Fax: 906-228-4421
E-mail: annconst@up.net

**Lisa Culver, PT, MBA**
Associate Director, Department of Practice

American Physical Therapy Association
1111 North Fairfax Street
Alexandria, VA 22314-1488
Phone: 703-684-2782 ext 3172
Fax: 703-838-8910
E-mail: Lisa Culver@apta.org

**Yanira Cruz-Gonzalez, MPH**
Director, National Council of LaRaza
1111 19th Street, NW, Suite 1000
Washington, DC 20036
Phone: 202-776-1745
Fax: 202-776-1792
E-mail: ycgonzalez@nclr.org

**Linda Dark, RN**
Project Manager, Division of Health Education
National Association for Equal Opportunity in
Higher Learning
8701 Georgia Avenue, Suite 200
Silver Spring, MD 20910
Phone: 301-589-5894
Fax: 301-589-8860
E-mail: Ldark@nafeohealthed.org

**Stephanie Dopson, MSW, MPH**
Health Communications Specialist
CDC/DDT
4770 Buford Highway, K-10
Atlanta, GA 30341
Phone: 770-488-5004
Fax: 770-488-5966
E-mail: SDopson@cdc.gov

**Mildred L. Freeman**
Director, Division of Health Education
National Association for Equal Opportunity in
Higher Learning
8701 Georgia Avenue, Suite 200
Silver Spring, MD 20910
Phone: 301-589-5894
Fax: 301-589-8860
E-mail: MFreeman@nafeo.org

**Pamela Garmon, MBA**
Marketing Manager, American Heart
Association
National Center
Dallas, TX 75231
Phone: 214-706-1650
Fax: 214-706-5233
E-mail: Pamela.Garmon@heart.org

**Julianna S. Gonen, PhD**
Director of Family Health
Washington Business Group on Health
50 F Street, NW, Suite 600
Washington DC 20001
Phone: 202-628-9320
Fax: 202-628-9244
E-mail: Gonen@wbgh.org

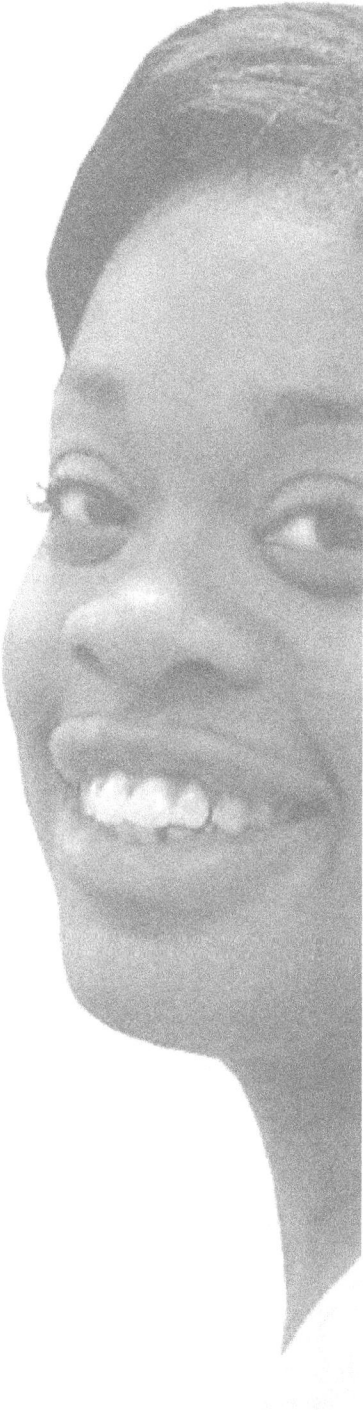

**John Graham, IV**
Chief Executive Officer
American Diabetes Association
1701 North Beauregard Street
Alexandria, VA 22311
Phone: 703-549-1500
Fax: 312-440-2800
E-mail: CMurray@diabetes.org

**Donette E. Green**
Manager
Health and Wholeness Program
The Congress of National Black Churches
2000 L Street, NW, Suite 225
Washington, DC 20036
Phone: 202-296-5657
Fax: 202-296-4939

**Yvonne Green, RN, MSN, CNM**
Associate Director for Women's Health, CDC
1600 Clifton Road, D-51
Atlanta, GA 30333
Phone: 404-639-7231
Fax : 404-639-7331
E-mail: Ygreen@cdc.gov

**Angela Green-Phillips, MPA**
Chief
Office of Policy and Program Information
CDC/DDT
4770 Buford Highway, K-10
Atlanta, GA 30341
Phone: 770-488-5028
Fax: 770-488-5966
E-mail: AGreen-Phillips@cdc.gov

**Barbara C. Hansen, PhD**
Lay Advisory Board Member
Juvenile Diabetes Research Foundation
6501 Bright Mountain Road
McLean, VA 22101
Phone: 410-706-3168
Fax: 703-356-4143
E-mail: bchansen@aol.com

**Sabrina Morris Harper, MS**
Senior Public Health Analyst, CDC/DDT
4770 Buford Highway, K-10
Atlanta, GA 30341
Phone: 770-488-5028
Fax: 770-488-5966
E-mail: SHarper@cdc.gov

**Barbara Hatcher, PhD**
Director
Scientific and Professional Affairs
American Public Health Association
800 I Street, NW
Washington, DC 20001-3710
Phone: 202-777-2490
Fax: 202-777-2533
E-mail: Barbara.Hatcher@apha.org

**Nancy Haynie-Mooney**
Health Communications Specialist CDC/DDT
4770 Buford Highway, K-10
Atlanta, GA 30341
Phone: 770-488-1153
Fax: 770-488-5966
E-mail: NHaynie-Mooney@cdc.gov

**Shelly Heath-Watson, MA**
National Director
Outreach Programs
American Diabetes Association
1701 North Beauregard Street
Alexandria, VA 22311
Phone: 703-299-2013
Fax: 703-253-4358
E-mail: SWatson@diabetes.org

**Marsha Henderson, MCRP**
Director
Office of Women's Health
Food and Drug Administration
5600 Fishers Lane, MS HF-8
Rockville, MD 20857
Phone: 301-827-0350
Fax: 301-827-0926
E-mail: Mhenders@oc.fda.gov

**Shannon Hills, MPA**
Marketing Manager—Women's Initiative
American Heart Association
National Center
7272 Greenville Avenue
Dallas, TX 75231
Phone: 214-706-1200
Fax: 214-706-5233
E-mail: Shannon.Hills@heart.org

**Nora Howley, MA, CHES**
Project Director
HIV/School Health Council of Chief State
School Officers
1 Massachusetts Avenue, NW
Washington, DC 10001-3700
Phone: 202-336-7033
Fax: 202-371-1766
E-mail: NoraH@ccsso.org

**Linda T. Jackson**
Director
Health and Wellness Program,
National Caucus and Center on Black Aged,
Inc.
1424 K Street, NW, Suite 500
Washington, DC 20005
Phone: 202-637-8400
Fax: 202-347-0895
E-mail: ltjacks@ncba-aged.org

**Jeannette Jordan, CDE**
National Spokesperson for African American
Nutrition, American Dietetic Association
304 Mulberry Drive
Summerville, SC 29483
Phone: 843-876-1949
Fax: 843-821-9373
E-mail: JordanJF@musc.edu;
Jeannette.Jordan@hcahealthcare.com

**Edith Kieffer, PhD, MPH**
Associate Research Scientist
Department of Health Behavior and Health
Education
University of Michigan School of Public
Health
1420 Washington Heights
Ann Arbor, MI 48109-2029
Phone: 734-647-2739
Fax     734-763-7379
E-mail   EKieffer@umich.edu

**Liz Kreese, MA**
Senior Staff Associate
Health Programs
U.S. Congress of Mayors
1620 I Street, NW, 4th Floor
Washington, DC 20036
Phone: 202-861-6756
Fax: 202-293-2352
E-mail: LKreese@usmayors.org

**Richard Levinson, MD, DPA**
Associate Executive Director for Programs and
Policy, APHA
800 I Street, NW
Washington, DC 20001-3710
Phone: 202-777-2443
Fax: 202-777-2532
E-mail Richard.Levinson@apha.org

**Meredith Lee, MPH**
Health Policy Analyst
American Public Human Service Association
National Association of State Medicaid
Directors
810 First Street, NE, Suite 500
Washington, DC 20002
Phone: 202-682-0100
Fax: 202-682-3706
E-mail: Mlee@aphsa.org

**Helen Leonard**
Program Coordinator
Society of State Directors of Health
Physical Education and Recreation
1900 Association Drive
Reston, VA 20191-1599
Phone: 703-476-3403
Fax: 703-476-0988
E-mail Hleonard@aahperd.org

**Norma Loner**
Committee Management Specialist, CDC/DDT
4770 Buford Highway, K-10
Atlanta, GA 30341
Phone: 770-488-5376
Fax: 770-488-5966
E-mail: Nloner@cdc.gov

**Peggy Mainor, JD**
Senior Advisory
Federal Relations Council
American Indian Higher Education Consortium
121 Oronoco Street
Alexandria, VA 22314
Phone: 703-838-0400
Fax: 703-838-0388
E-mail: Pmainor@aihec.org

**Kathy McNamara**
Assistant Director of Clinical Affairs
National Association of Community Health
Center
1330 New Hampshire Avenue, Suite 122
Washington, DC 20036
Phone: 202-659-8008
Fax: 202-659-8519
E-mail: KmcNamara@nachc.com

**Michael Meit, MA, MPH**
Director
Center for World Health Practices
University of Pittsburgh
116 Interstate Parkway
Bradford, PA 16701
Phone: 814-362-8656
Fax: 814-362-8632
E-mail Meit@pitt.edu

**R. Scott Mitchell**
Managing Editor and Webmaster for
CBCFHealth.org
Congressional Black Caucus Foundation, Inc.
1004 Pennsylvania Avenue, SE
Washington, DC 20003
Phone: 202-675-6733
Fax: 202-547-3806
E-mail: ScottMY98@aol.com;
Scott.Mitchell@cbcfhealth.org

**Saul Malozowski, MD, PhD, MBA**
Senior Advisor for Clinical Trials and Diabetes
Translation
Division of Diabetes
Endocrinology, and Metabolic Diseases
National Institute of Diabetes and Digestive
and Kidney Diseases
6707 Democracy Boulevard, Room 679
MSC5460
Bethesda, MD 20892
Phone: 301-435-9774
Fax: 301-480-3503
E-mail sm87j@nih.gov

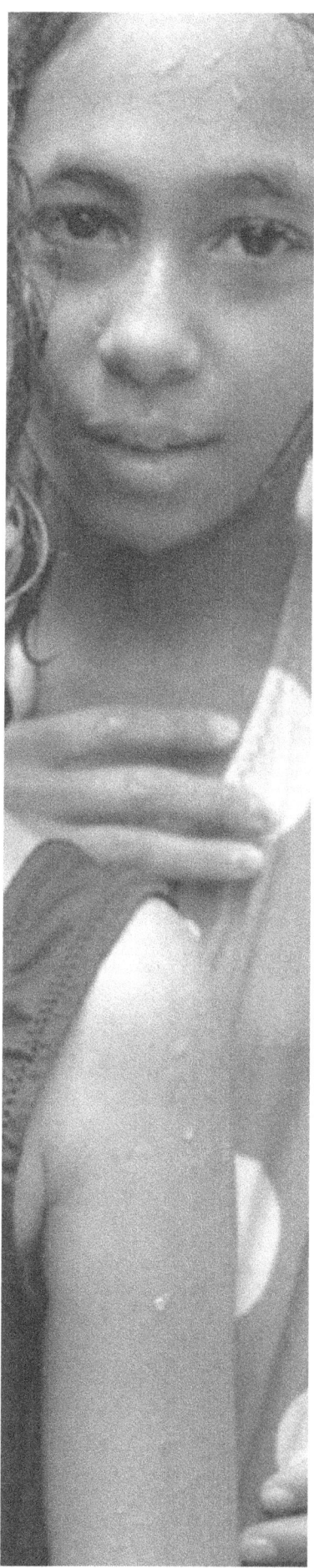

**Dara Murphy, MPH**
Chief
Program Development Branch
CDC/DDT
4770 Buford Highway, K-10
Atlanta, GA 30341
Phone: 770-488-5046
Fax: 770-488-5966
E-mail: DMurphy@cdc.gov

**Kathleen Nolan, MPH**
Senior Director
Prevention Policy
Association of State and Territorial Health
Officials
1275 K Street NW, Suite 800
Washington, DC 20005
Phone: 202-371-9090
Fax : 202-371-9797
E-mail: KNolan@astho.org

**Michelle Owens, PhD**
Team Leader
National Public Health
Initiative on Diabetes and Women's Health
CDC/DDT
4770 Buford Highway, K-10
Atlanta, GA 30341
Phone: 770-488-5014
Fax: 770-488-5966
E-mail: MOwens1@cdc.gov

**Elena Rios, MD, MSPH**
President
National Hispanic Medical Association
1411 K Street, NW, Suite 200
Washington, DC 20005
Phone: 202-628-5895
Fax: 202-628-5898
E-mail: NHMA@nhmamd.org

**Kathy Rufo, MPH**
Deputy Director
CDC/DDT
4770 Buford Highway, K-10
Atlanta, GA 30341
Phone: 770-488-5000
Fax: 770-488-5966
E-mail: KRufo@cdc.gov

**Susan Russell**
Staff Assistant
DHHS/Office on Women's Health
200 Independence Avenue, SW, Room 712E
Washington, DC 20201
Phone: 202-205-1952
Fax: 202-401-4005
E-mail: SRussell@osophs.dhhs.gov

**Saira Saeed, MPH**
Program Manager
Diabetes American Association of Health Plans

1129 20th Street, NW, Suite 600
Washington, DC 20036
Phone: 202-778-8478
Fax: 202-778-3287
E-mail: SSaeed@aahp.org

**Izzat Sbeih, MPH**
Health Policy Analyst
American Public Health Association
800 I Street, NW
Washington, DC 20001-3710
Phone: 202-777-2493
Fax: 202-777-2533
E-mail: Izzat.Sbeih@apha.org

**Karen Sherwood, MS, MBA**
Program Manager
Women's Health
American Association of Health Plans
1129 20th Street, NW, Suite 600
Washington, DC 20036
Phone: 202-778-8471
Fax: 202-778-3287
E-mail: KSherwood@aahp.org

**Kim Stratiou, RD**
Nutrition Program Coordinator
National Association of WIC Directors
P.O. Box 2448, Room 132
Richmond, VA 23218
Phone: 804-692-0001
Fax: 804-692-0223
E-mail: KStratiou@vdh.state.va.us

**Henrietta Terry, MS**
Program Analyst
DHHS/Office on Women's Health
200 Independence Avenue, SW, Room 712E
Washington, DC 20201
Phone: 202-205-1952
Fax: 202-401-4005
E-mail: HTerry@osophs.dhhs.gov

**Kristen Tertzakian**
Tobacco Control Policy Analyst
Association of State and Territorial Health
Officials
1275 K Street NW, Suite 800
Washington, DC  20005
Phone: 202-371-9090
Fax: 202-371-9797
E-mail: KTertzakian@astho.org

**Patricia Thompson-Reid, MAT, MPH**
Program Development Consultant
CDC/DDT
4770 Buford Highway, K-10
Atlanta, GA 30341
Phone: 770-488-5017
Fax: 770-488-5966
E-mail: PThompson-Reid@cdc.gov

**Susan Baker Toal, MPH**
Writer/Consultant
917 Barton Woods Road
Atlanta, GA 30307
Phone: 404-378-3256
Fax: 404-378-3256
E-mail: SToal@mindspring.com

**Frank Vinicor, MD, MPH**
Director
CDC/DDT
4770 Buford Highway, K-10
Atlanta, GA 30341
Phone: 770-488-5000
Fax: 770-488-5966
E-mail: FVinicor@cdc.gov

**Carol Watson, MPH**
Senior Project Director for Women's and
Perinatal Health
Association of Maternal and Child Health
Programs
1220 19th Street, NW, Suite 801
Washington, DC 2036
Phone: 202-775-0436
Fax : 202-775-0061
E-mail: CWatson@amchp.org

**Violet Woo, MS, MPH**
Health Policy Analyst
DHHS/Office of Minority Health
The Rockall 2 Building, Suite 1000
5515 Security Lane
Rockville, MD 20852
Phone: 301-443-9923
Fax: 301-443-8280
E-mail: VWoo@osophs.dhhs.gov

**Odette Wynter-Tuckson**
Associate Director
Outreach Programs
American Diabetes Association
1701 North Beauregard Street
Alexandria, VA 22311
Phone: 703-299-2064
Fax: 703-253-4358
E-mail: OWynter-Tuckson@diabetes.org

**Patricia Yarholar, MPH, CHES**
Diabetes Coordinator
Association of American Indian Physicians
1225 Sovereign Row, Suite 103
Oklahoma City, OK 73108
Phone: 405-946-7072
Fax: 405-943-1190
Email: Pyarholar@aaip.com

**Peggy Yen, RD, MPH**
Nutrition Consultant
Association of State & Territorial Public Health
Nutrition Directors
Department of Health and Mental Hygiene
Division of Cardiovascular Health
6 St. Paul Street, Suite 1202
Baltimore, MD  21202
Phone: 410-767-6781
Fax: 410-333-8926
Email: YenP@dhmh.state.md.us

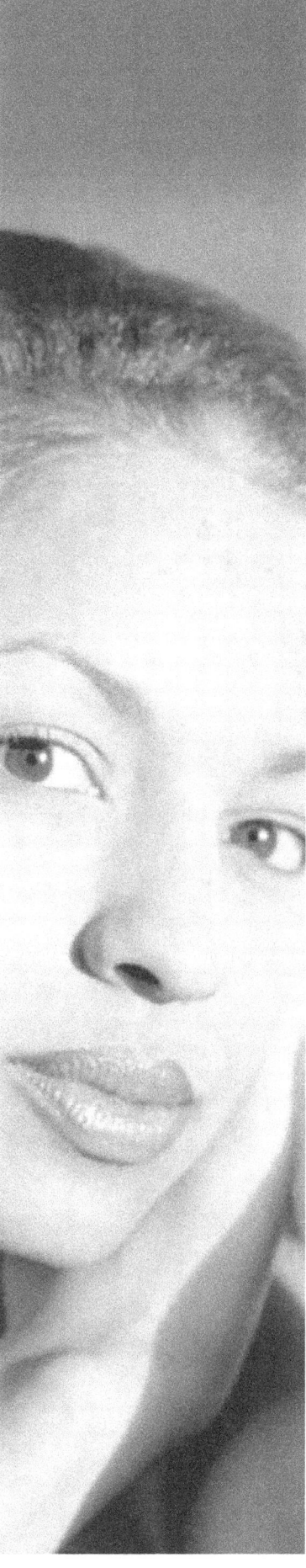

# APPENDIX B: REVIEWERS

**Ann Albright, PhD, RD**
Director
Diabetes Control Program,
California Department of Health

**Christopher Benjamin, JD, MPA**
Program Development Consultant
Division of Diabetes Translation
National Center for Chronic Disease
Prevention and Health Promotion
Centers for Disease Control and Prevention

**Barbara Bowman, PhD**
Associate Director for Policy Studies
Division of Diabetes Translation
National Center for Chronic
Disease Prevention and Health Promotion,
Centers for Disease Control and Prevention

**Charlene Burgeson, MA**
Public Health Advisor
Division of Nutrition and Physical Activity
National Center for Chronic Disease
Prevention and Health Promotion
Centers for Disease Control and Prevention

**Carl Caspersen, PhD**
Associate Director for Science
Division of Diabetes Translation
National Center for Chronic Disease
Prevention and Health Promotion
Centers for Disease Control and Prevention

**Magda Ciocazan, MPH**
Public Health Prevention Specialist
Division of Diabetes Translation
National Center for Chronic, Disease
Prevention and Health Promotion
Centers for Disease Control and Prevention

**Odette E. Colón, BFA, MFA**
Graphics Specialist in support of Office of the
Director, Information Resource Management,
Centers for Disease Control and Prevention

**Ana Alfaro-Correa, ScD, MA**
Program Development Consultant
Division of Diabetes Translation
National Center for Chronic Disease
Prevention and Health Promotion
Centers for Disease Control and Prevention

**Paula Duncan, MD**
Professor of Pediatrics
University of Vermont Medical School
Incoming President
American Academy of Pediatrics

**Michael Engelgau, MD**
Chief
Epidemiology and Statistics Branch
Division of Diabetes Translation
National Center for Chronic Disease
Prevention and Health Promotion
Centers for Disease Control and Prevention

**Christine Fralish, MLIS,**
Chief, Technical Information and Editorial
Services Branch
National Center for Chronic Disease
Prevention and Health Promotion
Centers for Disease Control and Prevention

**Linda Geiss, MA**
Chief
Surveillance Section
Division of Diabetes Translation, National
Center for Chronic Disease Prevention and
Health Promotion
Centers for Disease Control and Prevention

**Catherine Gordon, MD, MSc**
Assistant in Medicine and Instructor
Endocrinology/Adolescent Young Adult
Medical Practice
Eating Disorders and EndocrinologyPrograms
Harvard Medical School

**Regina Hardy, MS**
Assistant Branch Chief
Epidemiology and Statistics Branch
Division of Diabetes Translation
National Center for Chronic Disease Prevention
and Health Promotion
Centers for Disease Control and Prevention

**Carol Hinton**
President and Chair
State Adolescent Health Coordinators
Association

**David Hoffman, MEd**
Director
Bureau of Chronic Disease Services
New York State Health Department

**Rick Hull, PhD**
Writer Editor
National Center for Chronic Disease
Prevention and Health Promotion
Centers for Disease Control and Prevention

**Giuseppina Imperatore, MD**
Epidemiologist
Division of Diabetes Translation, National
Center for Chronic Disease Prevention and
Health Promotion
Centers for Disease Control and Prevention

**Jane Kelly, MD**
Director
CDC National Diabetes Education Program
Division of Diabetes Translation
National Center for Chronic Disease
Prevention and Health Promotion
Centers for Disease Control and Prevention

**Juliette Kendricks, MD**
Associate Director for Science
Division of Reproductive Health
National Center for Chronic Disease
Prevention and Health Promotion
Centers for Disease Control and Prevention

**Siri L. Kjos, MD**
Professor and Chief
Division of Women's Health
Department of Obstetrics and Gynecology
Keck School of Medicine
University of Southern California

**Qaiser Mukhtar, PhD**
Epidemiologist
Division of Diabetes Translation
National Center for Chronic Disease
Prevention and Health Promotion
Centers for Disease Control and Prevention

**Yolanda Sacipa, MPH**
Florida Diabetes Control Program
Representative
Florida Diabetes Control Program

**Arlene Sherman**
Management Information Assistant
Division of Diabetes Translation
National Center for Chronic Disease
Prevention and Health Promotion
Centers for Disease Control and Prevention

**Mary Kay Sones**
Health Communication Specialist
National Center for Chronic Disease
Prevention and Health Promotion
Centers for Disease Control and Prevention

**Jan Weingrad Smith, CNM, MS, MPH**
Assistant Professor
Nurse Midwifery Education Program
Boston University School of Public Health

**Quion Wilkes**
Office Automation Clerk
Division of Diabetes Translation
National Center for Chronic Disease
Prevention and Health Promotion
Centers for Disease Control and Prevention

**David Williamson, PhD**
Epidemiologist
Division of Diabetes Translation, National

Center for Chronic Disease Prevention and
Health Promotion, Centers for Disease
Control and Prevention

and Task Force Members

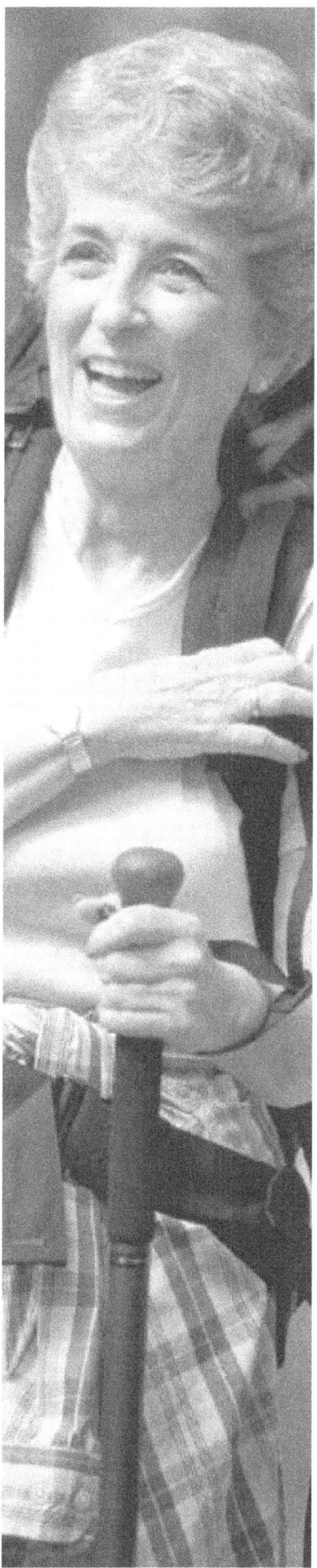

# APPENDIX C: REFERENCES

Beckles GLA, Thompson-Reid PE, editors. ***Diabetes and Women's Health Across the Life Stages: A Public Health Perspective***. Atlanta: U.S. Department of Health and Human Services, Centers for Disease Control and Prevention, National Center for Chronic Disease Prevention and Health Promotion, Division of Diabetes Translation, 2001.

Boyle JP, Honeycutt AA, Narayan KMV, Hoerger TJ, Geiss LS, Chen H, Thompson TJ. ***Projection of diabetes burden through 2050***. Diabetes Care 2001;24:1936-40.

Centers for Disease Control and Prevention. ***Socioeconomic status of women with diabetes: United States, 2000***. MMWR, February 22, 2002;51(07):147-8, 159.

Knowler WC, Barrett-Connor E, Fowler SE, Hamman RF, Lachin JM, Walker EA, Nathan DM. ***Reduction in the incidence of type 2 diabetes with lifestyle intervention or metformin***. Diabetes Prevention Program Research Group. New England Journal of Medicine 2002;346: 393-403.

Troiano RP, Flegal KM. ***Overweight children: description, epidemiology, and demographics***. Pediatrics 101(3) (Supplement to Pediatrics, Part 2 of 2):497-504, March 1998.

U.S. Bureau of the Census. ***Population Projections of the United States, by Age, Sex, Race, and Hispanic Origin: 1995 to 2050***. Current Population Reports, Series P25, No. 1130. Washington, DC: U.S. Government Printing Office, 1996.

U.S. Department of Health and Human Services. ***Healthy People 2010***. 2nd ed. With Understanding and Improving Health and Objectives for Improving Health. 2 vols. Washington, D.C.: U.S. Government Printing Office, 2000.

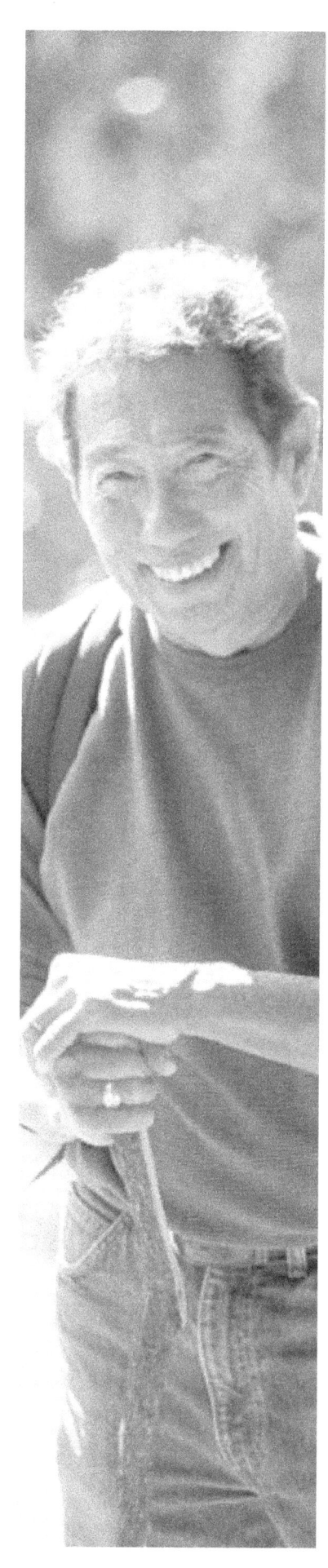

# CDC
# Division of Diabetes Translation
# Public Inquiries / Publications

**Phone Toll Free**:
1-877-CDC-DIAB (877-232-3422)
**Fax**:
301-562-1050
**Internet**:
www.cdc.gov/diabetes
**Email**:
diabetes@cdc.gov
**Mail**:
P.O. Box 8728,
Silver Spring, MD
20910

DEPARTMENT OF HEALTH AND HUMAN SERVICES
Centers for Disease Control and Prevention